RADICAL APPROACHES TO THE CARE CRISIS

Solidarity, Community and a National Care Service

Anne Gray

First published in Great Britain in 2025 by

Policy Press, an imprint of
Bristol University Press
University of Bristol
1–9 Old Park Hill
Bristol
BS2 8BB
UK
t: +44 (0)117 374 6645
e: bup-info@bristol.ac.uk

Details of international sales and distribution partners are available at
policy.bristoluniversitypress.co.uk

© Bristol University Press 2025

British Library Cataloguing in Publication Data
A catalogue record for this book is available from the British Library

ISBN 978-1-4473-7408-4 paperback
ISBN 978-1-4473-7409-1 ePub
ISBN 978-1-4473-7410-7 ePdf

The right of Anne Gray to be identified as author of this work has been asserted by her in accordance with the Copyright, Designs and Patents Act 1988.

All rights reserved: no part of this publication may be reproduced, stored in a retrieval system, or transmitted in any form or by any means, electronic, mechanical, photocopying, recording, or otherwise without the prior permission of Bristol University Press.

Every reasonable effort has been made to obtain permission to reproduce copyrighted material. If, however, anyone knows of an oversight, please contact the publisher.

The statements and opinions contained within this publication are solely those of the author and not of the University of Bristol or Bristol University Press. The University of Bristol and Bristol University Press disclaim responsibility for any injury to persons or property resulting from any material published in this publication.

Bristol University Press and Policy Press work to counter discrimination on grounds of gender, race, disability, age and sexuality.

Cover design: Namkwan Cho
Front cover image: Shutterstock/VLADGRIN

Contents

List of figures, tables and boxes		iv
List of abbreviations		vi
Acknowledgements		vii
Preface		viii
1	Introduction	1
2	Survey evidence on paid and unpaid care	16
3	How can informal care be sustained?	42
4	Who pays? How much care could be free, what kinds and for whom?	67
5	Widening the caring circle: towards a caring economy	94
6	Solidarity projects: mutual aid, timebanks, community unions and volunteers	118
7	Reducing the need for care	143
8	Conclusions and solutions	159
Appendix A: Cost calculations and revenue sources for expanding subsidised care		174
Appendix B: Seniors' different needs for help and how they are met		178
Appendix C: Stories of lived experience		183
References		191
Index		219

List of figures, tables and boxes

Figures

2.1	Time trend of informal carers as percentage of population and local authority spending on adult social care (England)	27
2.2	Trends in hours of informal caring per week, UK	29
3.1	Over-65s living alone, 1996–2019	48

Tables

2.1	Value of the care sector in England, 2018	19
2.2	Growth of homecare workforce compared to local authority homecare clients in England, 2015/16 to 2019/20	20
2.3	Trends in the number of informal carers in the UK	26
2.4	Use of formal and informal care by family type	35
2.5	Health Survey of England: need for help and unmet need among people over 65	36
2.6	Informal care by relationship of helper to the person being helped	39
3.1	Trend in number of childless women	50
8.1	The eight policy domains of 'age-friendly communities' and how community projects can contribute	172
A1	Possible sources of tax revenue to expand social care spending	175
A2	Cost calculation for homecare	176
A3	Estimated cost of residential and nursing care	177
B1	Help received and need for help, by age band	179
B2	Who helps with which tasks?	181

List of figures, tables and boxes

| B3 | Trend in contributions of different informal helpers, 2011–2018 | 182 |

Boxes

2.1	Survey questions about informal care	22
2.2	Caring from childhood	23
2.3	Love and loss: caring for a disabled adult daughter	30
3.1	Margaret's story: friends may become the 'family' of the childless	49
3.2	Hyacinth: when children cannot support parents enough	51
3.3	What an intensive carer loses	60
3.4	Elfrida: when families need carer's leave	62
3.5	Examples of carer's leave policies	63
5.1	Themes from the Campsbourne Community Collective's exhibition on care	101
5.2	Selected comments on the qualities of carers and caring from the Campsbourne project exhibition	102

List of abbreviations

ADLs	activities of daily living
DBS	Disclosure and Barring Service
ELSA	English Longitudinal Study of Ageing
FPC	free personal care
FRS	Family Resources Survey
HSE	Health Survey of England
IADLs	instrumental activities of daily living
IPPR	Institute for Public Policy Research
MAGs	mutual aid groups
NEF	New Economics Foundation
NLW	National Living Wage
NHS	National Health Service
RVS	Royal Voluntary Service
UBI	universal basic income
UKHCA	UK Home Care Association
WBG	Women's Budget Group

Dates expressed with dashes represent periods of time, for example 2010–2020.

Dates expressed with slashes (for example 2011/12) represent financial years as used by UK public services for budget data (1 April to 31 March), or to represent periods during which some large surveys collect and present data.

Acknowledgements

The author is most grateful to several people who provided stakeholder interviews or information about their projects: staff of ACORN, the Equal Care Coop, Community Catalysts, Fair Shares, Haringey Circle, Lewisham Local, Rochdale Circle, and a special thanks to the community research team of the Campsbourne Collective.

Several people should also be mentioned with appreciation of their helpful comments at various stages of development of the book proposal and the text: Simon Duffy, Jude Fransman, Kerry Forsman, Jay Ginn, Jerome de Henau, Susan Himmelweit, Les Levidow, Gordon Peters, Vincent Tickner and Samantha Webb. Any errors remain entirely the responsibility of the author.

Also thanks to End Social Care Disgrace for permission to reproduce transcripts of parts of their YouTube video, and for including the author in their helpful online meetings about the need for carer support.

Thanks to the UK Data Archive for access to the data for the English Longitudinal Study of Ageing and the Health Survey of England.

Thanks to London South Bank University for having provided library access and software during the author's post-retirement period as an unpaid visiting research scholar, and for having hosted her previous research since 1999.

Thanks to Skills for Care for permission to reproduce part of a table in Chapter 2.

Preface

How this book came to be written

What promoted this work on social care? I began with a qualitative study of people engaged in befriending schemes both as volunteers and 'befriended' and with volunteers running older people's social clubs in a London borough (Gray, 2006). Then came a more statistical investigation of what creates 'social capital' for older people (Gray, 2009). From 2011, I turned to the lives of people in retirement housing, to the question of how social activities and tenants' groups could give residents a sense of neighbourliness leading to mutual aid, and a collective voice about their housing conditions and services (Gray, 2015; Gray and Worlledge, 2018). I also became involved in local campaigns to preserve the health service and improve social care in the London borough where I live. Helping to run a pensioners' group with both social and advocacy/campaigning roles offered many insights into the daily lives of seniors struggling with self-care and the care of relatives, illustrated within this book. I experienced the harsh realities of helping to arrange care for my partner's parents in the United States, which presented a severe challenge to their children living thousands of miles away. This is perhaps not untypical for many London residents whose children or parents live abroad. I witnessed among my personal contacts the trials of seniors facing the COVID-19 pandemic on both sides of the Atlantic, impeded during lockdowns from contact with relatives, and with many normal facilities for support and socialising unavailable.

Having research experience about older people rather than younger care-needers, I have chosen to focus here on the needs of seniors, while acknowledging that the most rapid increase in demand now facing UK local authorities is for care of people of working age. But several policy issues affect both age groups; for example, for better public transport, for accessibility in public places and for a more inclusive society generally. The younger disabled grow older, and thanks to medical advances their life expectancy is rising. Many seniors are caring for a disabled son or daughter. Lastly, local authority budgets for care for all adults are combined under the heading of Adult Social Care; the shortage of funds in these budgets affects all age groups and gives them common cause to struggle for change.

Anne Gray
September 2024

1

Introduction

The themes and purpose of this book

The central theme of this book is how to deal with the mushrooming demand for social care in Britain's ageing society. It addresses some issues about budgeting for a national care service, especially the challenges of reducing or lifting user charges while paying care workers adequately. It considers the potential shortage of *unpaid* care, and how community solidarity can help fill some important gaps in the care system.

The first part (Chapters 2 and 3) describes the care shortage and how it is likely to worsen in coming years. It emphasises the dependence of adult care on *unpaid* support from family and friends. This is so large that state services can never replace it all, so we have to find a way to provide enough of it for the growing share of the population who are very old and/or disabled. Care budgets have not kept pace with the rising number of very old people in poor health, nor the even more rapid increase in disabled younger adults. Some evidence of the effects in terms of service reduction is summarised later in this chapter. The shortage of local authority funds since the financial crisis of 2008/9 has induced rationing of council-arranged care to those in greatest need, with a rising proportion of clients paying for all or part of their care package. Many have started buying care privately, outwith council arrangements. Many more cannot afford care. Shrunken council services mean extensive unmet need. Unpaid carers are caring for longer weekly hours, taking them away from their paid jobs and causing stress and ill-health for many.

Several organisations have advocated a free national care service, in parallel with the free National Health Service (NHS) and inspired by the Scottish policy of free personal care. They include the Green Party, the Liberal Democrats, the Campaign for a National Care, Support and Independent Living Service (NacSILs), the National Pensioners' Convention, Independent Age (2020) and the Trades Union Congress.[1] It is argued that the political and moral rationale for free universal health care, established since 1947, should be extended to social care. This would help many who currently cannot afford to pay; and among those who can, it would provide equity between care-needers and people in good health. While an attractive long-term aim, a demand for universal free care raises many questions about affordability and priorities.

Chapter 4 examines the likely cost of care reform, the difficult choices about how much care should be provided, what kinds and for whom. It explores the huge challenge of funding enough care for people currently 'priced out' by council charges, especially if care workers are paid fairly and adequately to recruit and retain the workforce. However, it also suggests some ways to reduce the cost of care services, which can improve quality at the same time. Chapters 5, 6 and 7 propose some solutions to the problem that an adequate state care service is likely to take many years to achieve. These solutions are based on community solidarity to sustain unpaid care and support the many non-medical measures which can help people stay healthier for longer. They are inspired by the concept of the 'caring economy' developed by the Care

---

[1] See the following websites: Green Party, https://greenparty.org.uk/2024/06/24/you-can-judge-a-society-by-how-it-looks-after-those-in-need-says-greens-as-they-promise-20bn-social-care-package; Liberal Democrats, https://www.libdems.org.uk/news/article/our-plan-for-social-care; National Pensioners' Convention, https://www.npcuk.org/post/road-map-to-social-care; National Campaign for a Care and Support Service for Independent Living (later renamed End Social Care Disgrace), https://endsocialcaredisgrace.org/; Trades Union Congress (TUC), https://www.tuc.org.uk/research-analysis/reports/new-deal-social-care-new-deal-workforce; Independent Age, https://www.independentage.org/sites/default/files/2020-10/Report_Final.pdf

Collective (Chatzidikis et al, 2020) and described in Chapter 5, in which care is seen as a collective responsibility of family, friends, community and state working together, in democratic ways, with agency and voice given to care-needers.

A more detailed summary of each chapter follows.

Survey evidence on paid and unpaid care (Chapter 2)

Chapter 2 offers a statistical portrait of formal (paid-for) care and the far larger scale of informal (unpaid) care. It also measures need and unmet need, examining how receipt of formal and informal care varies between people with family to help and childless singles, showing for whom is there unmet need, and with what tasks.

To define the scale of care required at population level inevitably relies on national surveys which provide indicators of people's capacity for basic activities of daily living and the support they need for these. However, people do not need merely to cope with everyday functions like washing, dressing, making and eating meals, cleaning, shopping and getting to the doctor. They also deserve a quality of life with enjoyment, company and cultural stimulation, which depends on not becoming isolated or housebound.

The care system relies heavily on unpaid carers, mainly partners, adult daughters of seniors and, to a lesser extent, sons. Sometimes, however, it is the older parent, most often the mother, who cares for a disabled son or daughter, often for decades. Excessive loads have been placed on family carers as formal care has shrunk in recent years.

The current role of informal care and likely future challenges to expanding it (Chapter 3)

Chapter 3 considers whether the current scale of unpaid care can be sustained, leading to a discussion of how unpaid carers could be better supported, to sustain their crucial role. Family-based care, already stretched to breaking point, is unlikely to keep pace with growing needs given adverse demographic and socio-economic trends – the rising retirement age, rising employment rates of older women, smaller and more dispersed families, and the growing proportion of younger generations who are disabled. The care deficit will likely worsen over the next 15 years or so. Modelling of future demand for care services suggests soaring budget requirements in future years as the oldest age groups grow, particularly if there is any shrinkage of the 'propensity to care' among those of working age. Because of the rising ratio of seniors to working-age people, even if the 'propensity to care' of the younger ones stays constant, there will be proportionately fewer of them to help. Still greater budget pressures come from the rapidly rising demand for care services from younger disabled adults. Thus demand for formal services will grow faster than need, increasing the fiscal challenge of making widespread free care affordable.

To sustain unpaid caring requires much better support of family carers. Chapter 3 considers how to replace the Carer's Allowance with an income for caring work, as well as the need for respite care and carers' paid leave from employment. It describes some international examples of good practice which expose the inadequacy of UK provisions. A universal basic income could also encourage shorter working time, reducing stress for carers. It would also ease the worry for unemployed people about taking time off from job search to care for sick relatives.

A small percentage change in the 'propensity to care' would lead to a much larger percentage change in demand for paid-for services. While Chapter 3 examines the risk of informal care failing to keep pace with demand, Chapters 5 and 6 consider how a small increase in community solidarity could help to make a formal care budget go further and reduce care charges.

The likely cost of care reform, the challenge of adequate pay for care workers and options for reducing or restructuring charges, including universal free care (Chapter 4)

Chapter 4 examines the cost of formal care and the problematic trade-offs that exist between the scale and scope of services, their unit cost and the extent of subsidy for users. It deals with the budget for *all* adult social care, since eldercare must be provided alongside better support for younger disabled people, most of whom are even more dependent on subsidised services and often hard-pressed relatives.

This chapter attempts to introduce realism and practical detail into debates about a free national care service, highlighting the difficult choice between reducing charges and improving care workers' pay. Several estimates suggest that abolishing charges for a substantial part of existing services would not present a major fiscal challenge – but existing services serve too few people and pay care workers very badly. Optimists have estimated that free personal care along the lines of the Scottish model would be feasible with existing wage levels. One London borough has already led the way, and a second plans to do so in 2025. However, there are difficult choices about the number of clients who can be supported, for how many hours or for what range of needs. The need for better care workers' wages makes a vast difference to the funds required and the feasibility of waiving charges. Another major funding requirement is for better remuneration of *unpaid* carers, for whom the Carer's Allowance is inadequate both in scale and design.

Care competes with the backlog of other calls on state budgets, including health, education, childcare, public transport, social housing, cash benefits and the 'green transition'. The entire public sector faces funding difficulties because of slow economic growth, the 'cost of living' crisis and the challenge of climate change. While Appendix A suggests many ways of raising more revenue, the sums of money they yield are stretched in many directions.

Fortunately there are several ways to provide care more cheaply which also offer quality improvements. They cannot solve the care budget deficit, but they can reduce it somewhat. Chapter 4 discusses various forms of not-for-profit provision, which can be highly personalised and user-directed. Expensive and unpopular residential care could be used less, substituting alternatives such as extra-care housing and 'shared lives'. Costs per client can be contained by changes in how needs are identified and how support is commissioned, focusing on the precise kind of help people want, with emphasis on early intervention.

What care needs or tasks would it cover – is 'personal care' enough or always the most important? The Fabian Society Commission (Harrop and Cooper, 2023) questioned whether subsidies should be wholly focused on *personal* care. Should the priority be free care for the most severe needs, or extending the range of tasks and people covered even if that means keeping some charges? What share of the vast amount of *unpaid* care should be replaced? How much should be expected of family carers, in terms of the hours they spend caring and the tasks they can reasonably cover? How should increasing pay for underpaid care workers be balanced against reducing charges for clients? Could unit costs of providing care be reduced by turning to micro-enterprise or non-profit cooperatives? Or by providing better and cheaper alternatives to residential care?

Solidarity and community development, to sustain and develop unpaid support (Chapters 5 and 6)

Support from non-relatives is the major theme of Chapters 5 and 6. They address the key challenge of how to sustain and increase informal care, by widening the circle of people involved beyond the family. These chapters attempt to develop the vision of the 'caring economy' put forward by the Care Collective (Chatzidikis et al, 2020), the Women's Budget Group (2020), Dowling (2021) and Segal (2023), for integrating paid-for and unpaid care within a framework of solidarity, based on the strengths of the community. This means working to improve the quality and quantity of state-funded care provision while sharing unpaid support more widely as a community responsibility. Solidarity and the 'caring economy' vision needs to be mainstreamed into the care reform debate, along with activism around co-production and service-user control.

Support from friends, neighbours and community projects cannot share the intimate tasks of 'personal care' that fall to professionals, partners, daughters and sons. But it could go far in supporting care-needers and family carers in many other ways, some of which are just not provided by formal services.

Chapter 5 switches away from the quantitative perspective of the earlier chapters, to consider caring more as a personal relationship with important interpersonal and emotional aspects. This challenges the rigid and un-empathic forms of care offered by the largely privatised agencies and residential homes in recent years. The importance of qualitative and emotional aspects of care are illustrated through the voices of carers in a London community project, with their experiences of isolation and emotional stress.

Chapter 5 introduces a discussion of network theory and how people form supportive friendships. It evaluates the experience of specific community projects designed to help them do that, such as North London Cares and the Rochdale Circle. Avoiding loneliness and isolation is increasingly recognised as important for preserving health, and for helping people to build and sustain forms of support that can delay or reduce their need for formal services.

Chapter 6 examines specific forms of community solidarity projects for their potential contribution to sustaining informal care and support:

- mutual aid groups which developed during the COVID-19 pandemic both in the UK and the United States;
- the ACORN community union movement;
- experiences of timebanking, in the UK and internationally;
- the contrasting and more traditional approach of the NHS Volunteer Responder programme.

Projects like these can support two important goals of the 'caring economy': more non-profit provision and more unpaid support to individuals from friends, neighbours and volunteers. For individuals, they can help to meet needs which are often unsupported by formal services as care is 'rationed' to the most severe needs. While formal services are often limited to bedroom and bathroom tasks, non-relatives can offer support with home and garden maintenance, cooking, digital skills support, and helping people go out and socialise. Through collective action in community organisations, they can help to preserve and grow day centres, lunch clubs, community transport, seniors' clubs and social activities. They can support non-profit enterprises providing formal care, offering volunteers, client referrals and possibly a premises base. They can bring together different forms of support for isolated people and family carers, helping to identify individuals who lack family or formal support and signposting them to services.

'Solidarity' is envisaged here as a vehicle for advancing the inclusion of age-impaired or disabled people of all age groups. It is used here to describe practices and values of unpaid support for impaired individuals, for their carers, and for community projects that provide collective services for them. It encapsulates forms of helping others which are largely informal and unmediated by state agencies or charities, but which do not necessarily depend on established friendships. Some contrasts are made with conventional volunteering, which also has an increasing role and potential since the COVID-19 pandemic.

'Solidarity' and mutual aid are closely related concepts. Unlike charity or much formal volunteering, they make no rigid distinction between helpers and helped. This retains dignity, autonomy and self-expression for those receiving support. Mutuality, in the context of the mutual aid movement such as the groups that developed during the COVID-19 pandemic, does not convey an obligation to reciprocate for support received. Rather, those receiving help are encouraged to contribute to the collective effort if they can.

As traditionally used in trade union circles, 'solidarity' conveys the meaning of standing together for change; it is a politicised form of helping which seeks to remedy the problems that give rise to needing support. By analogy with unions working together to challenge poor pay or working conditions, it includes applying political pressure for better formal care, better financial support for unpaid carers, for more accessible transport and housing for disabled people, both seniors and younger, as well as for securing them greater respect and voice.

Reducing the need for care (Chapter 7)

Chapter 7 considers how the social and physical environment can reduce the need for formal care, by helping people remain healthier for longer. This is not just about medical treatment or personal choices like not smoking. It requires building on community and individual strengths to link together, in a preventive, 'early help' approach, all the resources we have in both formal and informal care, and policies to make neighbourhoods age-friendly and disability-friendly.

Chapter 7 discusses how to keep down the rising trend of demand for care, recognising that demand for formal care is highly sensitive to the health status of the population. This invokes the need for preventive health measures, to extend *healthy* life expectancy, reducing the span of years during which care may be needed. These include early help in the development of older age impairments, identifying strengths and resources people can draw on, and ensuring they have the right kind of support, with choice and flexibility. Solidarity projects can contribute much to this preventive approach.

Also important is an inclusive and disability-friendly social and physical environment that reduces barriers to daily living and social activities for those with impairments, and develops voice, agency and solidarity for them within their neighbourhood. The Age Friendly Communities movement offers some valuable examples of how to address, at local level, the barriers that disabled people and their carers face in everyday life, such as isolation, poor housing and poverty. Age-friendly and disability-friendly public transport, accessible design of public spaces and buildings all help people get about and remain connected to their friends and communities. Neighbourhood quality and design also influence people's social contacts. Illustrating how the solidarity projects described in Chapters 5 and 6 could fit together with these policies, Chapter 7 ends with suggestions of how formal care resources could be used most effectively within coordinated neighbourhood networks of paid and unpaid support.

A summary of main themes and recommendations (Chapter 8)

The last chapter presents four main strands of solutions to the care crisis:

- Expanding formal services to meet unmet needs, particularly for personal care, and make formal care more affordable by encouragement of non-profit forms of formal services which can offer higher quality, often at lower cost, than corporate providers. A gradual transition to free universal care could be achieved in stages.

- Sustaining informal care and growing it in line with the population in need. This requires widening the circle of informal carers through personal networks and community solidarity, to address isolation and increase forms of instrumental support which can support family carers and those who have none, complementing formal services and filling in gaps in the range of needs it covers. Reshaping of Carer's Allowance into a wage-like carer's income, and better carer's leave rights, would help to relieve stress for intensive family carers.
- Co-production of care services by users and professionals, working towards better care quality and embedding formal services into the culture of age-friendly, disability-friendly neighbourhoods. This goes with outcomes-based commissioning, which can draw on the strengths of care-needers and their communities.
- Reducing the need for care through preventive health measures, and through working towards a more inclusive, accessible and disability-friendly physical and social environment. Extending healthy life expectancy is a key element of solutions to the care crisis, although not a short-term one. Rather, it is a way of keeping down the growth of demand for care services in coming decades.

Hopefully policy makers and lobbyists will find some useful material about how to advance both a 'caring economy' vision and the 'age-friendly communities' agenda. Advocates of a universal care service will find food for thought about how the 'ask' should be defined and how it might be funded, including the scope of free care and charging reforms which could offer stepping stones towards it. Unpaid family carers have a huge role which formal services cannot replace, but their number is not keeping pace with growing needs. Their work needs to be sustained and recognised as real work, with entitlement to an income, better carer's leave from jobs, and greater support from the wider community.

Sources and approaches used in this book

The book combines quantitative and qualitative approaches, combining secondary sources, stakeholder interviews, the author's own analysis of large surveys and reflections on the lived experience of seniors observed from among friends, previous research and voluntary work. It is written for activists and campaigners, as well as for social work and care sector professionals and the academic community.

Statistical material is drawn from the published reports of the Family Resources Survey (FRS), and the author's analysis of data from the Health Survey of England (HSE) and the English Longitudinal Study of Ageing (ELSA). Much of the statistical analysis for this work was done during the COVID-19 pandemic, when data collection for major government-sponsored surveys was impeded by lockdowns and the situation was abnormal in several ways. For this reason, the data presented here on the use of care are mainly up to 2018, to show snapshots and trends in pre-pandemic 'normal' times, although the latest statistical releases of the FRS are used where available and relevant. The latest wave of ELSA, released in March 2024, has not been used since it came out rather late in the process of completing this book. However, the 2018–19 data from ELSA and from the HSE in Appendix B are unlikely to be outdated, since the FRS and the HSE show little change over the previous decade in the role played by relatives versus non-kin in provision of informal care. The latest HSE data on social care, from the HSE 2021, are not fully comparable with the data of 2018 due to methodological changes. (The HSE was not done in 2020 due to the COVID-19 pandemic.)

Appendix C provides a few portraits of individuals to illustrate some of the problems and strengths of carers and of seniors in need of support. These are referred to here and there in the main text.

Setting the scene: the effect of shrinking care budgets

The context of this book is the shortfall of resources which has hit social care services since the financial crisis of 2008/9. Although well documented elsewhere (Dowling, 2021; Humphries, 2022; Lloyd, 2023) it is worth noting some main elements and effects of the decline in subsidised support from local councils.

Adult social care budgets suffered savage cuts following the financial crisis of 2008/9, falling from 2009/10 by over 1.7 per cent per year in real terms, while demand for care rose (Ismail et al, 2014).

After its lowest point in 2016/17, overall funding was restored to the 2011/12 level by 2021/2. But budgets faced very rapid inflation in 2021–3 with most of the new money for health and care going to the NHS. Meanwhile, both seniors and younger disabled people grow in number – the over-65s by almost a fifth between the 2011 and 2021 Censuses. Net spending on over-65s' care by English local authorities was only £577 per head of the older population in 2021/2; less in real terms than in 2010/11 (NHS Digital, 2022: Table 18).

The result was a drastic reduction in services, even before the COVID-19 pandemic:

- From 2009/10 to 2013/14, the number of non-residential care packages provided by English local councils fell by 39 per cent (Davis et al, 2019).
- From 2016/17 to 2020/1, the number of over-65s receiving local-authority-arranged long-term care (both homecare and residential placements) fell 6.7 per cent, from 587,000 to 548,435 (NHS Digital, 2019).
- The number of people of all ages who were assisted fell 20 per cent between 2009 and 2015 (Holmes, 2016).
- By 2016 some councils were also reducing 'personal budgets' that clients use to choose and buy their own care (ADASS, 2016).
- In 2018/19, only a quarter of over-65s who made a request received some form of local authority social care. A quarter received no services while half were directed to other services including the NHS, benefits system, voluntary groups or home adaptations (NHS Digital, 2018).
- Many residential and nursing homes are closing due to low placement fees from councils, while 'self-funders' pay around 40 per cent more than local authorities do for residential placements (Competition and Markets Authority, 2017).
- A severe shortage of residential placements has arisen since 2010 (Age UK, 2019; Incisive Health, 2019), placing stress on family carers of those most in urgent need of formal care.
- Respite care has been reduced, with an 11 per cent drop in the number of carers getting a respite break compared to 2016–21 (House of Lords, 2021).

- Carer assessments for support fell from 450,000 in 2009/10 to 350,000 in 2017/18 (House of Lords, 2021).
- For both residential and homecare, local authorities fund a smaller share of clients each year as people's savings rise above the means test threshold of £23,250, which has been unchanged since 2010/11.

The COVID-19 pandemic stretched the care system more than ever. During January to March 2022, over two million hours of planned homecare could not be given due to lack of staff – with recruitment severely hampered by low pay (Samuel, 2022b). Three out of four members of the County Councils Network tightened eligibility requirements for subsidised social care in 2023/4; over half made some cuts in care services. Despite some injections of new money in 2020–4, the formal care system is still at breaking point. This exacerbates stress for family carers and the extent of unmet need especially among those who have no relatives available to help. It also means more people paying for all or part of their own care, both within council arrangements and independently of them.

As money runs short, around one-third of councils have leaned on family members to do more so that care packages can be cut. This is the latest stage of the longer-term problem of 'intensification of care', described in Chapter 2 – an increasing proportion of carers providing care for unsustainably long hours. The failures of the formal care system over the last 15 years have led to a dangerous dependence on increasingly stressed family members.

The shortage of local-authority-funded care, as well as years of delay in updating the means test, means more families paying towards care from their own resources. By 2016/17, only 35 per cent of users of homecare arranged by local authorities were entirely funded by their council; 45 per cent were self-funders and 11 per cent made a co-payment or 'top-up'. Almost 7 per cent of care recipients (of all ages), or their families, bought extra support for themselves outwith council arrangements (NHS Digital, 2018; Office for National Statistics, 2023a). The Health Survey of England shows that in 2011, two-thirds of over-65s receiving formal homecare had at least part of their package paid for by the local council, but by 2018 only a quarter did. The switch to privately funded care helps to explain why the care workforce has grown 8 per cent per year between 2012/13 and 2021/2. This substantial demand for care outside of local authority statistics reflects partly a desire for better standards than council contractors provide, but also a response to the tight rationing of subsidised care induced by austerity budgets. Those who cannot afford to pay remain in unmet need.

There is tension between the needs of different age groups. The greatest pressure on English local authorities care budgets is not from seniors but from the soaring demand from rising numbers of working-age disabled people. Their homecare needs are often more severe than those of seniors. They also more often need residential care. For example, over 21 per cent of those with learning disabilities live in supported housing or residential homes, compared to around 11 per cent of those over 65.[2] Of 1.8 million requests for care made to English local authorities annually, around 72 per cent are from over-65s; but these take only around half the budget. Unsurprisingly, where budget shortage leads to rationing of care, it is by need and by ability to self-fund. Those seniors who have had long, healthy working lives are likely to have savings. However, as advocates of the 'care cost cap' proposal have argued, these savings can be rapidly eroded in case of prolonged need for self-funded care, especially in residential placements.

Could local authorities have done better? In Scotland, spending and service levels have held up much better despite abolition of charges for the 'personal care' element from 2002. However, as described in Chapter 3, some areas have seen longer waiting times and cuts to other services, including day centres. In Wales, the number of seniors receiving care did not keep pace with population between 2006/7 and 2014/15, with no evidence that disability was decreasing (Holtham, 2018). A more generous means test than the English one was introduced in 2016, with a £100 cap on weekly costs of homecare, later raised to £120.

---

[2] For learning disabilities, see Nuffield Trust Report. https://www.nuffie ldtrust.org.uk/resource/adults-with-learning-disabilities-who-live-in-their-own-home-or-with-their-family; for over-65s, see Gray (2015) on sheltered housing and NHS Digital (2019).

Introduction

Despite this, from 2016 to 2018, the total number of over-65s supported by social care services fell by over 11 per cent, while the older population continued to rise. In London, Hammersmith and Fulham abolished charges for homecare in 2015. Tower Hamlets had a 'free homecare' policy from the 1990s to 2017, when it reintroduced charges due to cuts in government grant, and plans to end charges again in April 2025.[3] Let us hope these pioneers continue their policies, despite the difficult state of local authority finance.

Terminology used in this book

The American terms 'eldercare' and 'seniors' are preferred here, being less wordy than their UK equivalents, 'care of older people' and 'older people'. 'Seniors', meaning here people over 65, perhaps also conveys a much-needed connotation of respect. 'Frailty' has entered health service vocabulary to describe people weakened by the process of ageing, but some regard it as demeaning; 'age-affected' or 'age-impaired' are the preferred term here except when it seems important to follow health service terms. Care which is part of someone's job or self-employment is described as 'formal' care; that which is not, as 'unpaid' or 'informal' care. Volunteering through an organisation falls between the two. It is regarded as 'informal' in the FRS. However, ELSA includes help from organised volunteers in the 'formal' category, because their organisation and supervision carries a financial cost, and they sometimes receive travel or other expenses.

---

[3] Real, a Tower Hamlets disability support charity, https://www.real.org.uk/news/statement-on-abolishing-social-care-charging-in-tower-hamlets/ and personal communication from LB Tower Hamlets press office, April 2024.

2

Survey evidence on paid and unpaid care

Introduction

This chapter considers the scale of unpaid care, who are its givers and receivers, and how it meshes together with formal (paid-for) care. It examines the scale of formal care relative to informal (unpaid) care, ways of measuring the amount of unpaid care and the number of people involved. Unmet need for care is assessed from the English Longitudinal Study of Ageing (ELSA) and the HSE.

Evidence from the growth of the care workforce and from the HSE demonstrates an expansion of self-funded purchases of care services in recent years. But this has failed to fill the gaps left by shrinking council services; unmet need remains high. The volume of unpaid care is only being sustained because more people are caring for very long hours, leading to acute carer stress. Lastly, the chapter examines how the amounts of formal and informal care received vary by whether someone has a partner or children to help; and long-term trends in how informal eldercare is distributed between relatives and non-kin.

The definition of 'care', and what tasks and facilities should be included in any definition of the need for support, is a crucial one. Some issues about this have arisen in implementing the free personal care policy established from 2002 in Scotland. 'Personal care' means help with washing, dressing, toileting, eating and taking medications – largely what one might call 'bedroom and bathroom tasks'. The recently published Fabian Society report (Harrop and Cooper, 2023) argued that Scottish 'free personal care' is too narrow a definition of care needs, and that services to promote social inclusion and wellbeing should also be included – an issue to be discussed further in Chapter 4. This invokes the growing concern with loneliness and isolation among frail seniors, which itself has significant consequences for health. Formal care for seniors, as currently delivered in England as well as Scotland, is concerned mainly with personal care, while informal carers are much more likely to provide company, see to domestic tasks and gardening, and help people go out. In fact, one effect of Scottish free personal care may have been to free family members to support seniors in other ways, once relieved of the tasks that homecare workers do. This will be discussed in Chapter 3.

The relative scale of formal and informal care

Unpaid care dwarfs the scale of formal care, but may not be sustainable over time as the responsibility becomes progressively more concentrated in fewer hands. The homecare industry has grown rapidly in recent years, but a large share of its services is purchased privately, not arranged through local authorities.

In money terms, estimating what it would cost as a paid service, unpaid care of adults of all ages was valued at £68.3 billion in 2016 (Office for National Statistics, 2017). The value can be measured through the 'household satellite accounts' developed by the Office for National Statistics to measure unpaid economic activity, and last calculated for 2016. By 2019, the National Audit Office estimated 'as much as £100 billion' (NAO, 2021). Carers UK (2021) put the value of informal care at £162 billion. Their estimate is based on 2021 Census data about the number of carers (including children who care) the hours for which they provide care, and the current value of care per hour. By comparison, UK local authorities plus the National Health Service spent only around £25 billion on social care for all adults in 2018, and a further £12 billion worth of formal care was privately purchased (Table 2.1). The National Audit Office (NAO, 2021) quotes a Laing-Buisson report that for over-65s alone, £1.5 billion was spent privately on homecare and supported living in England in 2018–19 and £6.8 billion on care homes.

Another way to examine the relative scale of formal and informal care is through the numbers of people engaged. The homecare industry employed a mere 560,000 workers in England in 2019/20, compared to the Census-based estimate of 4.75 million informal carers in 2021. Only around three per cent of over-65s in private households in England received formal care from home-carers, reablement staff or personal assistants in 2018/19, or 11 per cent if help with housework (usually from private cleaners) is included as well as personal care.[1] This compares to around eight per cent who, according to ELSA, had *informal* 'personal' care. The informal care additionally covers a wider range of tasks; 15 per cent received informal help with some *other* activity, including going out, shopping, cleaning and paperwork.

Scottish provision of state-supported formal care is far better than England's. In 2018, around 2.5 per cent of over-65s in Scotland received wholly state-funded homecare[2] under the policy of free personal care, compared to less than one per cent in England.[3] With free personal care, over 15 per cent of Scottish seniors receive some form of state-funded formal care and support, compared to under six per cent in England. These percentages are wider than personal care; they include adaptations, telecare, housing support, day care, advice and residential care.

Because much homecare demand has not passed through local authority assessments, its scale is best assessed through the industry's estimates of care purchased, shown in Table 2.1. Self-funded homecare in England outwith council arrangements was over one-third of total homecare expenditure by all purchasers in 2015–16. The savings conditions of the means test remain

---

[1] English Longitudinal Study of Aging (ELSA) Wave 9; author's analysis of data provided by Oldfield et al (2020) through the UK Data Archive; and HSE; author's analysis of data provided by NatCen Social Research (2023) through the UK Data Archive'.
[2] Figures on home care in Scotland are from Scottish Government (2019b); on population from https://www.nrscotland.gov.uk/files/statistics/population-estimates/mid-18/mid-year-pop-est-18-pub.pdf
[3] Author's analysis of Health Survey of England Data (2018).

Table 2.1: Value of the care sector in England, 2018

	Publicly funded and co-funded, £ thous.	Self-funded expenditure, £ thous.	Total, £ thous.
Residential care	8,790	3,061	11,851
Nursing care	2,541	4,448	6,989
Homecare	4,562	2,442	7,004
Day care centres	421	100	521
Other services	6,938	1,975	8,913
Direct payments, or 'personal budgets'	1,770		1,770
Total	25,022	12,026	37,049

Source: Adapted from Skills for Care (2018)/ICF Consulting (2018)

unchanged since 2010/11; other elements are unchanged since 2015. This means many more people now pay for all or part of their council-commissioned care; these clients' care is included in the first column of Table 2.1. By value, the homecare sector has grown at 2.2 per cent per year since 2017 to reach £5.5 billion in 2022,[4] whereas local authority expenditure on social care as a whole shrank in real terms by four per cent between 2011 and 2019–20 (NAO, 2021). The homecare labour force has grown while the number of people provided with homecare by local authorities has fallen, as shown in Table 2.2. The scale of self-funded homecare is important, since it is a likely source of expanded demand for a free or more heavily subsidised public service. Many people who have eligible needs but fail the means test for subsidised care would then apply to local councils. Reducing charges could cause unexpected pressure on services from people switching out of private arrangements that are outwith the knowledge of council social work teams.

---

[4] IBIS World press release, https://www.ibisworld.com/united-kingdom/market-size/domiciliary-care/. Data on the value of the homecare industry are published by private actors and not available for all dates.

Table 2.2: Growth of homecare workforce compared to local authority homecare clients in England, 2015/16 to 2019/20

	2015–16	2019–20	Percentage change
Number of homecare workers	510,000	560,000	+9.8
Number of adults receiving homecare commissioned by local authorities	486,945	469,450	-3.6

Note: This covers workers in Care Quality Commission registered establishments.
Source: UKHCA (2021)

Just over 318,400 seniors in England are in residential or nursing homes (Office for National Statistics, 2023a) – or, if the same share of the population applies, around 360,000 across the whole of the UK. While providing enough residential and nursing care is crucially important, especially as the numbers of dementia sufferers rise, it is used by only a small minority of seniors, most of whom wish to avoid institutional care for as long as possible. The alternative of extra-care housing, currently used by less than 7 per cent of seniors (Gray, 2015), may reduce the need for higher-cost institutional care and provide residents with a better quality of life. Its expansion is advocated by the Fabian Society in its proposals for care reform (Harrop and Cooper, 2023). More will be said about this and other alternatives to residential care in Chapters 4 and 7.

Estimates of the number of informal carers

Care-giving can be measured either by asking carers or asking receivers of care. Several major UK government surveys estimate the extent of informal care given and received in private households. The ones used here are:

- ELSA Wave 9 (2018–19);
- the HSE from 2011 to 2018;
- the Census for England and Wales, 2011 and 2021;
- the Family Resources Survey (FRS), covering all of the UK, various dates.

These sources offer data on the numbers of carers and care hours provided or received. The data presented here from the Census and the FRS are about the numbers *providing* care (to anyone of whatever age) while the data presented from ELSA and the HSE are about over-65s *receiving* it.

The 'time window' examined here is mainly the 'decade of austerity', starting in 2011 after the major round of local authority budget cuts in 2010/11. This term is often used to describe the period when public finances were severely squeezed and many public services, especially those run by local government, suffered shrinking budgets. Where appropriate, some information is added from earlier years and from the COVID-19 pandemic period (2020–1) or the post-pandemic period up to 2023 if available by the time of writing. The long-term trends are most easily seen in the years *before* the pandemic period, which was clearly abnormal both for the population and for the data collection process.

What is defined as informal care, and what are its boundaries? The questions used in three major surveys are shown in Box 2.1. Care may be for many years, or for a few days or weeks to help someone through a temporary illness or difficulty. It comprises several task categories. One of the annual FRS reports (FRS, 2018) analysed how different kinds of informal care changed over the period 2005–16. Measured in hours, two categories remained constant: personal (clinical and nursing tasks) and practical (directed at activities like shopping, cleaning and help with going out). The 'practical' type of support is least likely to be accepted as part of a formal care request, but is easiest to delegate to non-kin. *Continuous care* (that is, where the person required round-the-clock attention) is the only category that increased over those 11 years of FRS data; over 87 per cent of unpaid caring *hours* are for 24/7 care. It falls especially to women, as reflected in the high proportion of women among those caring for over 50 hours weekly (Parliamentary Office of Science and Technology, 2018). Long-hours caring seems to have been a response to the cutbacks in formal care from local authorities, and possibly also to the rising number of disabled people in the population. Such very intensive and demanding support is the kind of unpaid care that is most difficult for families and friends to provide.

Box 2.1: Survey questions about informal care

Census of England and Wales, 2021

'Do you look after, or give any help or support to, anyone because they have long-term physical or mental health conditions or illnesses, or problems related to old age?'

Census of England and Wales, 2011

'Do you look after, or give any help or support to family members, friends, neighbours or others because of either:

- long-term physical or mental ill-health/disability?
- problems related to old age?'

Family Resources Survey (FRS): 2008/9 questionnaire

'In some households, there are people who receive help or support because they have long-term physical or mental ill-health or disability, (or problems relating to old age). (Show card about types of help.) Is there anyone in this household who receives any of these kinds of help or looking after? Does anyone give help? ... And how about people not living with you: do you/ (or does anyone in this household) provide any help or support for anyone not living with you who has a long-term physical or mental ill-health problem or disability, or problems relating to old age? (Show card for the types of help to be included.)'

YouGov survey for Carers UK, 2020

'For the following questions, by "unpaid support", we mean helping someone who could be finding it hard to manage because of mental or physical illness, needing extra help as they grow older or because they have a physical or learning disability. This could be for anyone that you know (e.g. family, a friend, neighbour, colleague etc.).

Your support might include shopping, helping to find or arrange care or support, helping with managing money, giving regular emotional support, helping with transport, picking up prescriptions or providing hands on care (e.g. help with bathing, dressing etc.).' (Carers UK, 2020a)

Looking at provision of care for all adults, surveys vary in their estimates of how many unpaid carers there are in recent years. For England and Wales, the Census showed five million carers in 2021, some as young as five (see Burçu's story, Box 2.2 and Appendix C). To estimate the number of *adult* carers, one can deduct around 136,000 children under 17 according to Census data, although the Children's Society,[5] using a 2018 BBC survey, suggests 800,000. The Scottish government estimated 839,000 adult carers in September 2020.[6] Adding 219,600 for Northern Ireland (NISRA, 2022) brings the UK total to over 5.9 million adult carers in 2020–1. But the FRS finds only 4.2 million, although the number reached a higher peak of 5.6 million in 2012/13.

Box 2.2: Caring from childhood

> I think it's right that I start by saying that I did not know that I was a carer. How am I meant to know when I have been doing it since a young age? How am I supposed to know, when I am a child? How am I meant to know when I have not known any different? How am I supposed to know when this is my normal?
>
> In my case I guess it's more complicated when my parents didn't know any English ...
>
> But why didn't the GP say anything when a child accompanied their parent and translated? Why didn't the nurses notice when we visited my mum in hospital after school? I really hope that things have improved. (More of Burçu's story is in Appendix C)

---

[5] https://www.childrenssociety.org.uk/what-we-do/our-work/supporting-young-carers/facts-about-young-carers, p 3.

[6] https://www.gov.scot/publications/scotlands-carers-update-release-2/

One source of these variations is sample selection; the Census covers all residents, and the FRS a representative population sample. Another source of varying numbers is questionnaire differences (Box 2.1). Possibly the FRS question, which is prompted by a list of specific tasks, leads people to define their caring role more narrowly than the Census question. Carers UK has used YouGov polling annually for its Carers' Week Reports. In 2020 it covered 4,000 people representative of the general public, and by 2024 it had 6,000. It includes caring for disabled children (unlike the Census and FRS questions) and leaves out the mention of 'long term' conditions. YouGov revealed a much larger number of unpaid carers, estimated at 8.8 million in 2019, and nine million in 2020 just before the COVID-19 pandemic (Carers UK, 2020a). They found 4.5 million newly taking on some form of help for disabled or older people during the pandemic, sometimes just for shopping or emotional support – an important and encouraging finding which is discussed further in Chapter 6.

Carers UK also conducts its own surveys, using an online questionnaire to which people are invited to respond, defining care however they wish. With over 11,000 respondents in 2023, this survey provides valuable qualitative information about the challenges carers face. The sample is self-selected, being publicised among the organisation's members, affiliates, campaigners, volunteers, previous survey respondents, and through promotion among its employer networks, on social media and the Carers UK website. Respondents include carers of seniors, carers of younger disabled people and of disabled children. According to Carers UK (2021), this sample includes more women, and more carers doing very long hours, than there are in the overall population of carers identified in the Census or the FRS. This is probably at least partly because it includes carers of disabled children, who often require very intensive care, but the Census and the FRS ask about care for people who need it just because of their condition, rather than because they are young children.

Another reason why estimated numbers vary so much is that carers may count as 'caring' activities that the recipient defines as a family or friend visiting, or as the cooking and cleaning that 'naturally' falls to women. Conversely, not all carers think of themselves as carers, at least not at first (see Box 2.2).

The conceptual boundaries of *time spent* on care are elusive. When estimating care time, informal carers may, or may not, include travel time, keeping an eye on someone while doing childcare, housework or sleeping while 'on call'. Where the carer and the cared-for person share a household, extra housework, cooking or shopping may fall to the carer's lot but not actually be defined as caring. Empathy or family obligation may prevent an informal carer from thinking about care as 'work' or as competing with other activities (Bowes et al, 2019). But carers frequently reduce hours of paid work, often with serious financial consequences (Carers UK, 2023a, 2023b). The number of hours of caring per week is not the only measure relevant to carer stress. At least as important for carers may be interruptions, the sense of being 'on call', unable to rest or schedule other activities.

Trends in informal care compared to trends in need

As the share of seniors in the population grows, demand for care tends to grow faster than the resources available to provide it – unless the health of people in their final years can improve. During 2011 to 2021 the number of people over 65 in England and Wales grew by one-fifth, to over 11 million. But the total population grew only 6.1 per cent. The over-85s alone grew by 36 per cent, from 1.25 million to 1.7 million. This oldest group are the age group most likely to need eldercare; over 55 per cent had a disability in 2021 compared to around 27 per cent of those in their late 60s. While not all people with disabilities need care – some people can manage without and may not even want help – this does show how increasing life expectancy increases demand for support (Office for National Statistics, 2019, 2023a). An important goal is to help people to enjoy more years of *healthy* life expectancy.

Local authority care became more and more difficult to obtain during the 'decade of austerity', as annual budgets failed to keep pace with the rising number of adults needing care. Spending hovered at or below £25 billion between 2012/13 and 2018/19, although it rose during the COVID-19 pandemic (Figure 2.1). One might have expected the number of informal carers to rise in response; but both the FRS and the Census show that it

Table 2.3: Trends in the number of informal carers in the UK

	2011	2021	Percentage change 2011–21
Census			
No. of informal carers	6.5	5.9	-9.3
Percentage of adults providing care	11.4	9.0	
Family Resources Survey			
No. of informal carers	4.9	4.2	-14.0
Percentage of adults providing care	10.5	8.3	

actually fell (Table 2.3). The FRS shows a continued slow fall in the *proportion* of the population caring since 2010/11, with merely some brief interruptions to this trend (Figure 2.1). In earlier years (2003/4 to 2008/9) it was even higher, reaching over one in ten compared to seven to nine per cent since 2010. According to the HSE, the proportion of over-65s needing help who actually *received* unpaid help fell from 38 per cent to 31.5 per cent between 2011 and 2018. However, the HSE shows a larger and sustained number of adults of all ages providing informal care than the FRS or the Census – around 17 per cent in both 2011 and 2019 (Health Survey of England, 2021). The difference may be due to the way the question was asked. As mentioned earlier, both the FRS and the Census ask about *regular or ongoing* caring for people with long-term problems, then how many hours they do in an 'average week'. But the HSE asks if someone gave any help in the last month. Many more people can say they gave *some* than those who help regularly over a longer period.

The picture of what happened to informal care during and since the pandemic is somewhat unclear. This will be remembered as a period of extreme difficulty. Most day centres and respite care facilities closed. New residential placements were difficult to arrange, and people were afraid to enter them in case they were infected. Hospitals were overloaded, so that delays in admission caused great dependence on informal care. Establishing new arrangements for homecare became more difficult as homecare

Figure 2.1: Time trend of informal carers as percentage of population and local authority spending on adult social care (England)

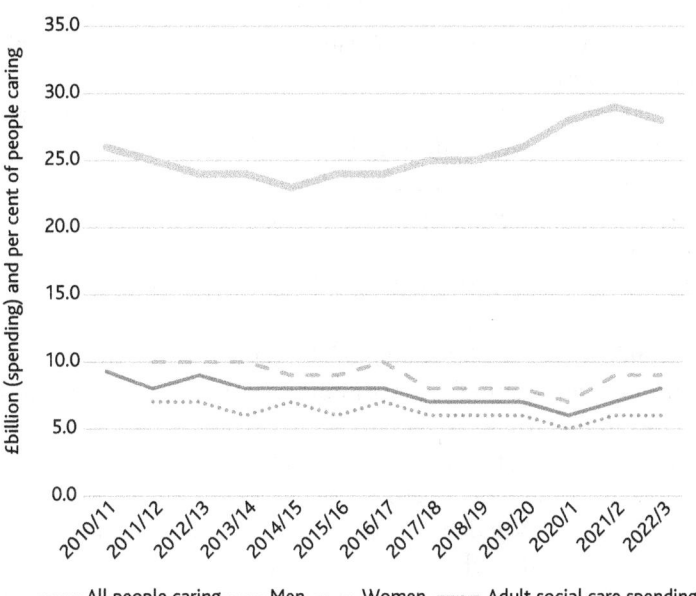

Notes: Spending data is in 2023 prices. Gender of carers is not shown for 2010/11 because of some changes in data availability. 2020/1 was an abnormal year because of COVID-19 pandemic restrictions on visiting.

Sources: Family Resources Survey (2018 and other years); King's Fund (2024a). https://www.kingsfund.org.uk/insight-and-analysis/data-and-charts/key-facts-figures-adult-social-care#how-much...?

agencies faced high rates of staff sickness and increased recruitment difficulties. Many families changed care arrangements during the pandemic, shifting responsibility from formal carers or visiting relatives to the care-needer's partner, as lockdowns and illness impeded visits by relatives outside the household. YouGov polling carried out for Carers UK (2020b) found a huge number of new informal carers during the lockdown period; but it is unclear how many of these were temporarily *replacing* those who normally provided it. The FRS, by contrast, shows a *drop* in informal care in 2020–1. Probably many of the new carers were temporary, standing in for arrangements that had been disrupted. The extra load on household members led to a huge increase in carer stress. The Association of Directors of Adult Social Services (ADASS, 2022a) reported that many family carers could not cope and made urgent requests for support. A large backlog built up of people waiting for care assessments. Some of the most helpful services to stressed informal carers, such as day centres and respite care, had been reduced severely during the period of austerity. Since the surviving ones closed during lockdowns, not all have re-opened.

There is a risk that long waits for assessment may push a carer over the edge of safety. In April 2022, the Association of Directors of Adult Social Services (ADASS, 2022b) reported that waiting lists for assessments had grown by 37 per cent since the previous November, to 542,000 people of all ages, of whom over 13 per cent had been waiting over six months (Samuel, 2022a). Among seniors, Age UK put the proportion much higher, at 28 per cent.[7]

When lockdown eased, the proportion of adults caring rose back to pre-pandemic levels, as shown in Figure 2.2, though not to 2011 levels. Whether this 'bounce-back' is sustainable is so far hard to tell. Although the very high weekly hours per carer of the pandemic period fell back, almost half of all carers were still doing over 20 hours per week. Many carers will have suffered overload for months. They may also be affected by long COVID or other health conditions that emerged or worsened when the pandemic impeded timely treatment.

Informal care left to fewer hands: the intensification of care and its impact on carers

A significant longer-term cause of carer stress is the trend to 'intensification of care' observed in both the FRS and the Census in recent years. This is the term often given to the rising proportion of informal carers who provide care for long hours. It is seen alongside a slight fall in the proportion of all adults in the population providing any informal care. Figure 2.2 shows trends in caring hours from 2012/13 to 2022/3, with the earlier comparison year of 2007/8. Average hours of informal care

---

[7] Age UK press release, 6 March 2023, https://www.ageuk.org.uk/latest-press/older-people-are-often-waiting-far-too-long-for-the-social-care-they-need/

Figure 2.2: Trends in hours of informal caring per week, UK

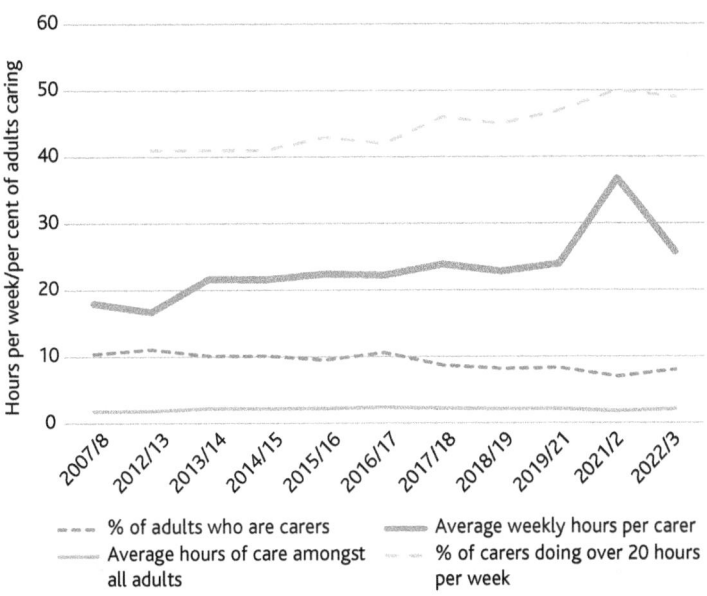

Notes: The years 2019–21 have been averaged to smooth the effects of the COVID-19 pandemic. Data on the percentage doing over 20 hours per week are unavailable for 2007/8.
Source: Family Resources Survey (2018 and other years)

provided, per adult in the UK population, remained constant only because of a rise in average hours per carer, from 17 hours in 2012/13 to 23 hours in 2018/19. The percentage doing over 20 hours per week rose from 41 to around 45. Thus a few people providing many more care hours per week compensated for the slight fall in the number doing any. There was a reduction in the lower 'tail' of people providing only a few hours per week (House of Commons Research Briefing, 2024). During the pandemic weekly hours per carer soared; afterwards, almost half of all carers still do over 20 hours per week.

A similar trend to intensification of care over the pre-pandemic decade is shown in the Census data. By 2021, half of those providing care did over 20 hours per week, compared to only one-third in 2011, and many more people were providing over

50 hours per week (Petrillo and Bennett, 2023). Long hours caring reached a peak as responsibility shifted to resident carers, mainly partners, during the pandemic; some visiting restrictions remained when the 2021 Census was taken in April. But the shift of informal eldercare from their children to partners is a much longer-term trend, as will be discussed in Chapter 3. Intensification may also be due to the shortage of subsidised formal care, combined with rising numbers of both dementia sufferers and disabled younger adults.

Intensification is particularly marked among older partner-carers. The 2021 Census shows that people in their late 70s and 80s are the most likely to provide over 50 hours of care per week. Many of these oldest carers have a long-standing illness or disability. Mostly they care for their partners, but sometimes for disabled sons and daughters, which may continue for decades (see, for example, Jo's story, Box 2.3).

Box 2.3: Love and loss: caring for a disabled adult daughter

I care full time for my 44-year-old daughter. I didn't ask for it or volunteer. The task is painful, but so filled with love. It's stressful, physically and mentally. It both isolates and creates new and unexpected friendships. ... I became a carer quite late in my life, compared to many of my caring colleagues. I was enjoying a very rewarding career. ... My youngest was a graduate student in London, enjoying her life to the full. She started to feel unwell, put her studies on hold and came home. Within ten months she was unable to move or speak, and received all her medication and food through a tube. A devastating neurological illness, caused by the measles virus, had ravaged her brain. That was 19 years ago. Since then ... I'm her prime carer and her dad is the support, and we've received a modicum of care worker support. (Jo's story; more in Box 3.3 in Chapter 3, and in Appendix C)

One priority for any expansion of free or subsidised services must surely be to relieve those who have the longest caring hours, especially if they are of working age or have health and care needs themselves. Brimblecombe et al (2017) surveyed unpaid carers together with care recipients of all ages; two-thirds of the carers said they needed more services, especially to free them for paid work. Even among the care recipients (who may not have fully appreciated the carer's need) almost half said they needed more services.

Carer stress

The lengthening of caring hours, reaching a peak during lockdowns, has had considerable impact on family carers. Successive surveys by Carers UK evidence the extreme difficulties they faced during the pandemic, exacerbating the problems many of them had for years before: isolation, lack of money, lack of any break from caring and even sufficient time to attend to their own health needs.

Support for the very old is obviously not the only demand on informal carers. A growing proportion of unpaid care during 2011–18 has been for younger people, according to the FRS for 2018. Just as local authorities are facing increasing demands on adult care services from those of working age, so the younger age group is needing more support from parents, siblings and friends. While disability prevalence among those of pension age fluctuated around 42 to 46 per cent in the last decade, the percentage of younger adults (16 to 64) with a disability rose from 16 in 2011/12 to 19 in 2019/20. It then jumped to 23 per cent in 2021/2, showing the severe effects of the COVID-19 pandemic on mental health (House of Commons Research Briefing, 2023). At the same time the proportion of *children* who are disabled has risen from six to eight per cent between 2011/12 and 2019/20, with a further upturn since the pandemic, partly due to mental health issues. Not only is formal support in short supply, but families are struggling to cope, sometimes with helping two generations of relatives needing disability support at once. Compounding the rising ratio of seniors to working-age adults, more younger people are becoming *care-needers* rather than able to provide care, although some set aside their own difficulties to help older relatives nonetheless.

For informal carers of working age, caring often competes with their need to maintain paid work. Many informal carers face financial hardship associated with being unable to do enough paid work, and a risk of ill health (Carers UK, 2023b,

2023c). The FRS in 2021/2 showed that out of all informal carers, half provided 20 or more hours per week, and 38 per cent over 35 hours. Only half had paid work, 22 per cent were retired, and 13 per cent were of working age but sick or disabled, leaving 15 per cent who may have been prevented from paid work by caring.

Research studies vary about how many hours people can spend caring in a week without having to leave or downsize a paid job. Aldridge and Hughes (2016) put it at 20 hours. Some other researchers have put the threshold at ten hours weekly (King and Pickard, 2013). Aldridge and Hughes found from the FRS that among working-age people caring for at least 20 hours weekly, 27 per cent were in poverty, compared to only 21 per cent of non-carers. Among working-age carers providing over 20 hours care per week, only 28 per cent manage full-time employment, while 16 per cent work part-time and over half do no paid work. Around 13.6 per cent of over-65s across the UK do paid work (Office for National Statistics, 2022) and seniors may face awkward decisions about whether to retire early or abandon pension-boosting earnings to look after their partner.

Carers lose out on pensions, promotion and career prospects (Carey et al, 2018). They often lack time to take sufficient exercise, to have a social life, to see about their own medical treatment, or even to organise a healthy diet. This affects their mental and physical health; many suffer stress and depression. Responsibility for eldercare falls more to adult daughters than sons, compounding the issues mothers face about access to paid work, promotion, training and pensions. Daughters are 27 per cent of unpaid helpers, according to the HSE 2018, while only 17 per cent are sons.

How formal care varies with the presence of an informal carer

Table 2.4 shows the proportions of seniors receiving formal care by partnership status and whether they had children. Formal help is heavily concentrated on single people. Among those with difficulties of daily living, between 4 and 5 per cent of couples have formal help, including cleaners, as do around 11 per cent of un-partnered people.

The concentration of formal care resources on single people mirrors considerable reliance on partners to reduce the formal care requirements of seniors in couples. This raises the question of how willing partners are to provide care, and how long the oldest among them (sometimes in their late 80s or even 90s) can sustain it. In addition to the stress faced by intensive carers of any age, older carers may wonder how far, and for how long, their own physique can manage helping someone who is increasingly unable to move around the home unaided. If the cared-for person is the heavier of the couple, helping them in and out of bed or in the bathroom may be nigh on impossible for the partner. Even pushing a wheelchair for someone heavier than yourself may be a major challenge on slopes or when entering a small lift.

The guidance given to local authorities about the Care Act 2014 laid down that having an unpaid carer should not affect assessment of need. Crucially, the initial 2014 guidance emphasised the willingness of the carer:

> 10.21. In considering the person's needs and how they may be met, the local authority must take into consideration any needs that are being met by a carer. The person may have assessed eligible needs which are being met by a carer at the time of the plan – in these cases the carer should be involved in the planning process. Provided the carer remains willing and able to continue caring, the local authority is not required to meet those needs. However, the local authority should record where this is the case in the plan, so that the authority is able to respond to any changes in circumstances (for instance, a breakdown in the caring relationship) more effectively. (Department of Health and Social Care, 2014)

The current guidance, under review in September 2024, (Department of Health, 2024) says:

> 10.26. Local authorities are not under a duty to meet any needs that are being met by a carer. The local authority must identify, during the assessment process,

those needs which are being met by a carer at that time, and determine whether those needs would be eligible. But any eligible needs met by a carer are not required to be met by the local authority, for so long as the carer continues to do so. The local authority should record in the care and support plan which needs are being met by a carer, and should consider putting in place plans to respond to any breakdown in the caring relationship.

The 2024 guidance makes several references to the needs of the unpaid carer, but seems to make assessment of the crucial concept of 'willingness' dependent on the carer's assessment being carried out:

> 6.18 … where the local authority is carrying out a carer's assessment, it must include in its assessment a consideration of the carer's potential future needs for support. Factored into this must be a consideration of whether the carer is, and will continue to be, able and willing to care for the adult needing care. (Department of Health and Social Care, 2024)

Long waits for assessment, and a shortage of respite care or day services, obviously increase the risk of carer 'burnout'.

Seniors with a resident partner are much less likely to have formal care, as shown in Table 2.4. However, having adult children does not seem to make a difference. Possibly there are two alternative effects of the presence of adult sons and daughters. One is to increase the use of formal care if children help to arrange it, or even pay for it. Alternatively, the children may offer more informal care instead, especially if formal care has to be self-funded. Much obviously will depend on how far away they live.

The measurement of need and unmet need

As an indicator of the extent of need, and what tasks people need help with, both surveys and Care Act assessments

Table 2.4: Use of formal and informal care by family type

	N	Percentage of family type with ADL/IADL difficulties	People over 65 with ADL/IADL difficulties			Formal help
			Informal help			
			Average hours of informal help per week*	Percentage who get informal help		Percentage who get formal help
Partner and children	832	25.5	13.5	57.6		4.4
Partner, no children	73	23.6	12.5	56.2		5.5
Children, no partner	527	39.0	7.8	54.6		11.0
No partner, no children	101	34.1	2.2	27.7		10.9
All family types	1533	29.3	10.8	54.3		7.2

Note: * Calculated on 'banded' hours data, over all cases in the row whether they actually receive any or not so that no informal help counts as zero.

Source: English Longitudinal Study of Ageing (ELSA) Wave 9; author's analysis of data provided by Banks et al (2024) through the UK Data Service

consider difficulties with 'activities of daily living' (ADLs) and 'instrumental activities of daily living' (IADLs). ADLs are eating, bathing, dressing, getting in and out of bed, using the toilet, and walking across a room, while IADLs include food shopping, housework, meal preparation, managing money and taking medication. The Care Act 2014 states that formal care should be offered to those who need help with two or more outcomes, corresponding to specific ADLs or IADLs, where this has a significant effect on their wellbeing. The concept of wellbeing covers many aspects of life which go beyond the basic physical functions captured in the ADL and IADL indicators. Loneliness, difficulty going out or maintaining the home and garden are also major issues, but largely unaddressed by formal care. Later chapters will deal with how these gaps might be filled.

For each ADL or IADL, ELSA and the HSE ask whether a person has difficulty with that task, then whether s/he receives or needs help with it. Age UK makes annual estimates from ELSA of unmet need, defined as those who have insufficient support for one or more ADLs that they can't manage without help. The number has grown steadily, by 2019 reaching over 1.4 million, or 14 per cent of over-65s (Age UK, 2023). The HSE uses a wider definition; someone has unmet need if s/he lacks help for any single ADL *or IADL* that s/he cannot do alone without difficulty (Dunatchik et al, 2016). Table 2.5 shows that the share of HSE respondents having needs for support with ADLs or IADLs fell slightly from 2011 to 2018, and so did unmet need. Fortunately, seniors' health had improved slightly during this period. Despite this improvement, unmet need according to the HSE definition remained at 24 per cent of seniors who had ADL or IADL difficulties.

The need for care rises with age and is higher for women, partly because more women survive into their 80s. In the HSE 2018, 30 per cent of women, but only 19 per cent of men, said they needed help with *two or more* ADLs or IADLs.

Table 2.5: Health Survey of England: need for help and unmet need among people over 65

	2011			2018		
	All	Men	Women	All	Men	Women
	(%)	(%)	(%)	(%)	(%)	(%)
Needed help with any ADL	32	27	36	24	22	31
Needed help with at least one ADL but received none	26	21	31	24	19	28
Needed help with any IADL	13	11	15	11	10	12
Needed help with at least one IADL but received none	16	14	17	13	12	15
N	1,676	757	919	1,798	1,064	1,188

Source: Author's analysis of HSE

As free council homecare has shrunk, private purchases have risen. The HSE shows that in 2011, 8.8 per cent of seniors with some ADL or IADL difficulties had some homecare paid for by their local authority, while 3.5 per cent bought some homecare privately. In 2018, only 3.1 per cent had any free council care, but almost 12 per cent bought privately.

Help with ADLs and IADLs is not all people need; they may also experience loneliness, isolation, poverty or poor housing. Several of the 'outcomes' specified in the Care Act as measures of wellbeing refer to the person's need for travel, social participation and relationships. It would be possible, even common, for someone to say 'I have no difficulties with ADLs or IADLs' yet still be badly in need of company, cultural stimulation or exercise. Loneliness is increasingly recognised as a significant source of decline in the psychological wellbeing, physical health, memory and cognition of seniors (Nyqvist and Forsman, 2015). ELSA measures the extent of loneliness in several ways, and also asks about access to a vehicle or to lifts. It would be interesting to know what people get lifts for – just for shopping or medical appointments, or also to visit friends, a library or cultural events?

ADLs and IADLs mainly define physical rather than social needs. ELSA's questions about care wanted and received cover *food* shopping. But dignity, wellbeing and self-confidence may be affected by lack of ability to access things *other* than food – like clothes, toiletries, books or hairdressing. Garden and home maintenance are not on the list of 'difficulties' but may significantly affect wellbeing. Seniors cannot always afford contractors; nor indeed, in a period of considerable excess demand for construction workers, can they easily obtain paid help with little things which a younger household might manage for themselves, like mending a garden gate or draught-proofing an ill-fitting window.

Seniors also need help with using the internet. This really needs to be listed as a separate item of need, so ubiquitous is the requirement to carry out online transactions with banks, local council, utility companies, tax and benefit offices, and retailers. Lack of skills or confidence, or of access to a suitable device or broadband connection, eyesight problems, dexterity and memory problems, are all problems some seniors face about doing things online. Around one-fifth of seniors cannot use the internet, while many more lack crucial competences (Age UK, 2024).

The providers of informal care: partners, children, other relatives and non-kin

Partners are the main source of informal care, as shown in Table 2.6. This raises the question of how caring affects an ageing partner's wellbeing. Is she/he strong enough to cope and for how long? Carers UK point out that 9 per cent of carers are over 75 (Carers UK, 2022). Conversely, Age UK in 2023 found that one in three people over 80 are carers.[8] Some care for grown children, rather than their partner (see Jo's story in Boxes 2.3, 3.3 and Appendix C).

Partner care is a fragile arrangement, depending so much on the partner's survival and fitness. In the over-65 age group, ELSA for 2018–19 (Wave 9) shows more men care for women (55 per cent) than vice versa (44.4 per cent), contrasting with women's predominance among younger carers. But as couples age, the dominance of women helping men re-emerges; among those over 85, 62.7 per cent of help from partners is women helping men.

The group of seniors most at risk of having no informal care are the childless singles. They are 6 per cent of the 5,225 people over 65 in the ELSA sample. Unsurprisingly, those with no partner are more likely to have difficulties that suggest a need for care; because they are older, they are mainly widowed. Unfortunately, the sample size is too small to analyse receipt of care by age group *within* each family type. Estimates based on the HSE (Brimblecombe et al, 2018) show that in 2014–16, 12 per cent of the five million people *providing* informal eldercare were partners who were themselves over 65, and 2 per cent were younger partners.

Average hours of informal help per week are much less for childless singles than for those with a partner or children. This is

---

[8] Age UK press release, 19 December 2019, https://www.carersuk.org/press-releases/carers-uk-reacts-to-age-uk-research-showing-over-80s-provide-23-billion-of-unpaid-care/

Table 2.6: Informal care by relationship of helper to the person being helped

	Percentage of those with ADL or IADL difficulties who are helped by this type of helper	No. of helpers shown in the survey	Percentage of these helpers who gave help in the last week	Average hours of help provided in the last week*
Spouse/partner	56.0	757	92.6	22.6
Daughter	28.8	389	84.3	9.8
Son	22.3	301	82.7	9.3
Grandchild	8.6	116	78.4	4.9
Sister	3.3	45	75.6	9.1
Brother	1.5	20	70.0	3.1
Other relative	4.4	60	71.7	3.4
Friend	12.6	171	77.2	3.9
Neighbour	3.8	52	61.5	1.7

Note: * Where respondent says this person sometimes helps, but not last week, this is counted as zero.
Source: ELSA Wave 9, 2018–19, author's analysis of data provided by Banks et al (2024) through the UK Data Service

despite single seniors being more likely to need help, since the risk of both widowhood and ADL/IADL difficulties increases with age. Over a third of single seniors have such difficulties, compared to under a quarter of those in couples. If someone has children, they tend to replace the partner as the main carer as the caring parent ages and eventually dies. Sometimes there is help from others beyond the immediate family circle. But more distant relatives and non-relatives do less caring per week; only 5 per cent provided 20 or more hours. This makes people without close relatives far more dependent on formal care. However, Table 2.4 shows that the percentage of single seniors receiving formal care is merely 11 per cent of those with ADL or IADL difficulties – not enough to compensate for the lack of help from partners.

As people lose their partners, daughters take over; they are the main category of informal helper for those over 84, and the second largest category after partners for the 75–84 group. In the ELSA

Wave 9 sample of over-65s who have ADL or IADL difficulties, almost 29 per cent are helped by daughters and 22 per cent by sons, either gender offering on average between nine and ten hours help per week. Across all parents over 65 with ADL or IADL difficulties (including people whose children don't help at all), couples receive on average 1.5 hours help per week from their children, and unpartnered seniors six hours. Friends and neighbours do appear to offer more help to seniors without available relatives. Almost a quarter of unpartnered seniors without children got help from non-kin, but only 6.2 per cent of couples did.

Siblings and grandchildren, step-grandchildren and other relatives play a much smaller role than adult children, helping only 6.4 per cent of seniors who have children and 7.1 per cent of those who don't. Non-relatives played a larger role, helping 16.4 per cent of seniors. By contrast, the FRS shows non-relatives as only 7 per cent of helpers for care-receivers of *all ages*. The likely reason for the difference is that care-receivers under 65 include many disabled adults helped only by their parents. This raises the issue of who will care for these people when their parents pass away.

Conclusion

This chapter highlights the predominance of *unpaid* or informal care, and the trend towards more formal care being self-funded in recent years. However, the amount of informal care and the number of unpaid carers are hard to measure, with great variation between different estimates. Unmet need for care among seniors remains high despite a slight improvement in their health during recent years. Neither formal care nor unpaid care has kept pace with the increase in life expectancy, which, sadly, often means surviving longer but in poor health. This results in intensification of care; the proportion of unpaid carers who are supporting relatives for very long hours is increasing, while the total number of carers is falling. Carer stress is rising, and more people experience conflicts between caring and maintaining paid employment. The heaviest loads are taken by parents of disabled sons and daughters who are unable to live independently. But seniors have also become the main carers for their partners; the role of adult children in informal care has diminished since the 1990s.

People without partners or children have the greatest care deficit. Less than 28 per cent get *any* informal help, receiving on average only 2.2 hours per week. They do get more formal care, but not enough to compensate, so that seniors with neither partner nor adult children are especially likely to experience unmet need. Even for seniors with partners, much of the partner-care offered may be unsustainable as the strength and health of either one declines. Their children face an increasingly difficult labour market to reconcile with parent-care.

The next chapter considers how the unpaid care deficit, particularly for single or childless people, will evolve over time.

3

How can informal care be sustained?

Chapter 2 has shown how the total volume of informal care has been sustained only by becoming more concentrated in fewer hands, causing much stress. This 'intensification' of care is due partly to unpaid carers replacing shrunken council services, but it is also rooted in several longer-term social and demographic factors.

This chapter deals with future trends in need, to highlight a growing gap that family care may not be able to meet. The need for care will rise by almost two-fifths up to 2040, and there are many reasons why informal care may not keep pace. These include the rapid relative growth of the oldest age groups, declining family size, labour market factors and the rising rate of disability among younger generations. Support of younger disabled people is in fact the most rapidly rising element in local authorities' caseload. All these factors underline the case for expansion of formal care. They also pose the twin challenges of how to ease carer stress, while sustaining and expanding informal care to keep up with growing need. This means developing better support services and financial help to family carers. It also invokes the question of how to share informal care more widely, which is the subject of Chapters 5 and 6.

Women have the greatest responsibility for informal care, which compounds their existing disadvantage in the labour market. Mothers are the most frequent carers of disabled adult sons and daughters, although among retired couples, men are slightly more likely to give care to women than vice versa. Some households have care needs for two generations at once, with care of both parents and disabled sons or daughters falling mainly to women.

There is an important gender dimension to receiving care as well as giving it. Although women do more caring than men over their life course, they are more likely to face unmet need in older age when it comes to their own care. This is because they tend to live longer than men, and once widowed, their children will be their main informal carers – if they have any. Having a partner or children to help is thus very important for women, who are also more likely to have activities of daily living (ADL) and/or instrumental activities of daily living (IADL) difficulties than men. The HSE's published report for 2021 shows that 28 per cent of women, but only 24 per cent of men, needed help with at least one ADL. Intensive caring is a health risk, which affects women more than men.

Also addressed in this chapter is the 'substitution debate'; the question of whether unpaid care is likely to fall in response to a greater offer of subsidised formal care. This is reviewed with reference to the Scottish experience since 2002, when free personal care (FPC) was first introduced there for seniors.

Four trends affecting supply and demand for informal care

Overall changes in the ratio of those needing care to those potentially able to provide it arise mainly from four trends:

1. the ratio of older people to working-age adults;
2. the incidence of disability among seniors;
3. the incidence of disability among people of working age, and to a lesser extent among children;
4. changes in the 'propensity to care'; the proportion of the population who are able, available and willing to provide informal care.

The fourth trend is the most complex. It is affected by the rising state pension age, the employment rate of women, the balance of care provision between partners, sons and daughters, and the willingness of non-kin to offer care. Finally, carer stress places a most important constraint on the propensity for unpaid care. Ways to ease this stress involve policies for carer support, from the state and from employers.

The growing care deficit due to population ageing

The UK population share of over-65s in the UK population will rise from 19 per cent in 2022 to 22 per cent in 2032 (Centre for Ageing Better, 2022). The need for care increases with age. Unless there are substantial health improvements among the very old, much more care will be needed by people over 85 whose number is expected to double between 2021 and 2040.

Thus the demand for care, especially formal care, is very sensitive to changes in the proportion of seniors who have disabilities or long-term health conditions. The later the age at which disabilities begin in older age, the lower the demand for support with them will be (Ovseiko, 2007). If *healthy* life expectancy could be extended by three years, demand for care would actually fall, and if by only two years, demand would not rise between 2020 and 2040. Preventive health measures, aiming to prolong healthy life expectancy, are thus a key part of resolving the care shortage. As well as reducing smoking and alcohol consumption, healthy living initiatives may crucially include encouragement to maintain physical activity and social networks, which in turn increases the potential for seniors to support each other. These issues will be revisited in Chapter 7, on the theme of how to reduce the need for care by keeping healthier for longer.

The effect of demographic trends on adult care demand and informal care supply has been extensively modelled in recent years by the Personal Social Services Research Unit, later located at the London School of Economics and Political Science as the Care Policy and Evaluation Centre. In several papers, they have identified a likely shortage of care, both formal and informal, up to the later 2030s (Comas-Herrera et al, 2006; Pickard, 2015; Hu et al, 2020). The shortage reflects the increasing proportion of very old people who are more exposed to difficulties of daily living. Even if formal care provision expands in line with the number of over-65s in the population, informal care needs to expand in line with it too. The 2020 paper estimates that this requires a 45 per cent increase in informal care of ageing parents from their children by 2038, and doubts whether this is achievable. The ratio of people over state pension age to working-age adults is predicted to rise to 37 per cent by 2040 (taking into account that the pension age will rise to 67 during 2026 to 2028; Office for National Statistics, 2019).

Another paper from the same research team (Brimblecombe et al, 2018) estimated that given rising life expectancy, and if the prevalence of disability within each age band remained constant, the number of over-65s in England needing care would increase from 2.1 million in 2015 to 3.5 million in 2035. Even if the proportion of these who actually received *formal* care also remained constant – unlikely, unless far more government funding is provided – the number of informal carers for seniors would need to rise by over three-fifths to 8.1 million in 2035. Much of this would be provided by partners, hopefully through a rise in male life expectancy. But because the younger population is growing more slowly than the over-65s, the total number of potential carers would only reach 5.85 million by 2035, leaving a shortfall of almost 2.3 million informal carers. The expected scale of this shortfall assumed the proportion of carers in the population, in each category by age, gender and relationship to the care-needer, would remain constant. But as shown in Chapter 2, the volume of unpaid care, in terms of hours provided, is maintained only because total care hours are becoming more unevenly shared, with rising strain and poverty among those who do very long hours. Sustaining the 'propensity to care' requires more people to take part.

Similar assumptions to those of Brimblecombe et al (2018) were made in a projection of supply and demand for informal care by Hu et al (2018). Over the period 2015 to 2040, they expected the number of seniors needing help with ADLs or IADLs to rise by over two-thirds, from 3.5 million to 5.9 million. To ensure that a constant proportion of those needing care would receive formal services, local authorities would need to provide care for 87 per cent more seniors in 2040 than in 2015. They would need to take over some clients currently buying care privately, because private care would become even less affordable as its cost tends to rise faster than pensions. Given that factor, help from their children would need to rise by 60 per cent.

These projections raise grave doubts about whether the 'propensity to care' can be maintained. The stress on some family carers, especially partners of seniors and parents of disabled adults, is unsustainable, and so is the impact on their ability to earn money, especially for those below pensionable age. This calls for more financial and other forms of support to encourage unpaid carers and wider sharing of caring responsibilities.

Care from partners or from children?

The trend for partners to replace care from seniors' children

A long-term trend from the late 1980s onwards for partner carers to replace adult children is one factor behind the 'intensification' of care described in the last chapter. Partners' role in eldercare has been increasing relative to that of daughters, sons and other informal carers (Hirst, 2002, 2005; Pickard, 2002, 2015). This reflected a fall in adult children living with their parents, when they often provided very long caring hours. According to the General Household Survey, 7.3 per cent of disabled over-65s received care from their partners in 1985 (Wanless, 2006). By 2022, the proportion rose to 22.5 per cent (Comas-Herrera et al, 2006). Children did continue to provide care to their parents, but more from their own separate households and for a lower number of weekly hours.

The HSE shows that the proportion of seniors with ADL difficulties who received care from their partners stabilised at 26 per cent between 2011 and 2018. That period saw some resurgence in the role of adult children, as shown in Table B3 (Appendix B). The percentage of seniors in need of help who received care from daughters rose from ten to 22 and from sons five to 14. Although a hopeful sign, it does not help the rising proportion of seniors without children.

There was a corresponding fall in very intensive care by partners. According to the Family Resources Survey (FRS), in 2011/12, almost one in five carers over 65 across the UK did more than 50 hours per week – a larger proportion than for any other age group. By 2019/20 only 16 per cent did so. Petrie and Kirkup (2018) note that although over one-fifth of sons and daughters who help their parents are involved only with IADLs, there has been a rise in the proportion helping with ADLs such as washing and dressing, especially since 2011/13. This was the period when social care budgets failed to keep pace with the growth in need.

The care deficit for lone childless seniors

In future there are likely to be more lone seniors without partner support, predominantly women. The absolute number of over-75s living alone in England and Wales has been rising since the 1990s (Figure 3.1), largely due to increasing life expectancy. This has been despite a falling *proportion* of older people living alone in each of the over-65 age bands, between the Censuses of 2011 and 2021. Successive age-cohorts of older women have become more likely to live with a partner (Crawford and Stoye, 2017), because more men are surviving into very old age, reducing the risk of widowhood. However, the trend for male life expectancy to catch up with female seems to have stalled or even reversed; men's median age at death rose from 78 in 2000 to 82 in 2010,[1] but fell back to only 81.8 by 2020. This may be partly to deficiencies in state health and care services.

Offsetting the fall in widowhood is an expected increase in people who enter their older years without a partner. In the 45–64 age group, the number of people who never married or are divorced rose 53 per cent between 1996 and 2017, compared to previous cohorts in England and Wales (Petrie and Kirkup, 2018). As this cohort moves into retirement, the proportion of single seniors will rise, making them potentially more dependent on other relatives or friends, or on formal care. Living alone not only reduces the chances of receiving informal care; it is also associated with poorer mental as well as physical health (Age UK, 2024a).

The trend in childlessness

Seniors without partners usually turn to their children for informal care; one-fifth of people over 85 rely entirely on their children

---

[1] ONS Census release, https://www.ons.gov.uk/peoplepopulationandcommunity/birthsdeathsandmarriages/lifeexpectancies/articles/mortalityinenglandand wales/pastandprojectedtrendsinaveragelifespan and earlier releases in the same series.

Figure 3.1: Over-65s living alone, 1996–2019

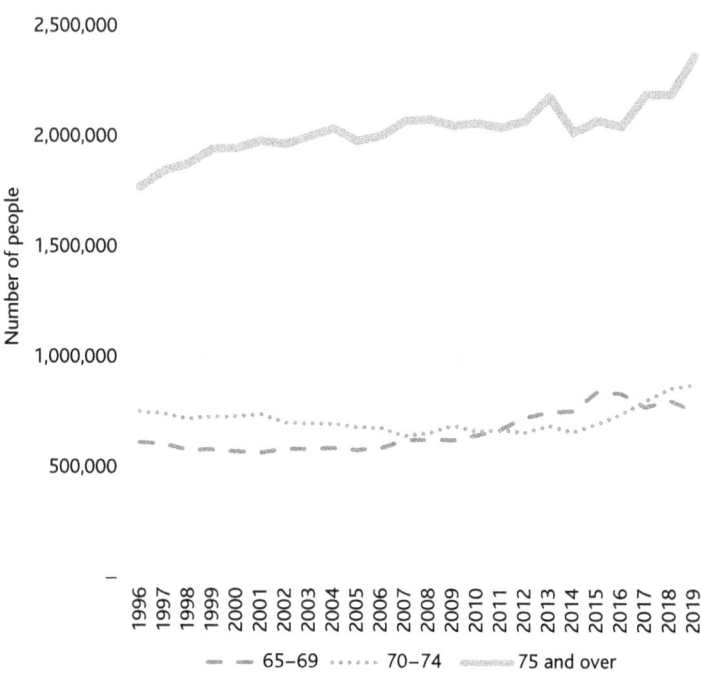

Source: Office for National Statistics (2020a)

(Office for National Statistics, 2020a). This raises the issue of what will happen to childless seniors in future years.

Almost one-fifth of women born in the 1970s – the ones now approaching retirement age – have no children. Table 3.1 shows how the proportion of childless women has changed over recent decades. Childlessness spiked for the generation born just after the First World War, who suffered the Second World War in their early 20s and reached 80 in the early years of the 21st century. Then it fell for those born in the 1940s and 1950s, but started rising again for those born in the 1960s and reached almost one in five for the 1970s cohort. Thus there will be a higher proportion of childless 80-year-olds in 2030 than at any time since 2000. Some seniors will find help from other sources – like Margaret, whose experience is related in Box 3.1. Others may not know enough able and willing friends.

Box 3.1: Margaret's story: friends may become the 'family' of the childless

Margaret, aged 71, lives alone and has no children. Shortly after moving home, she broke her leg by falling downstairs. Her split-level flat was being refurbished around her; works and mess were everywhere, with the upstairs bathroom stripped out. When she returned from hospital, her neighbours had moved her bed downstairs so she could use the lower bathroom, and had everything ready for her. She would have had to self-fund a carer, and had none; the hospital did not offer post-discharge carers. District nurses came to provide injections at first, but she had to struggle to get physiotherapy and found making repeated requests for this rather stressful. For several months she only left her flat when the ambulance crew carried her down a steep staircase and across a rough cobbled courtyard, to attend hospital appointments.

Margaret would have been lost without the many friends and neighbours willing to help her through the crisis. Fortunately, she knows many people through art workshops that she runs, through her choir, and former professional contacts. Friends visited by turns to prepare meals, stay with her and for the first few days empty her commode. The builders continued to work around her, and made her cups of tea. Supermarket delivery drivers often stayed to unpack her purchases into the fridge. Neighbours did other shopping and made sure she was OK; they know each other well, living in a gated development where people meet in the shared courtyard and car park, and through the leaseholders' management association.

Ageing Well Without Children[2] is an organisation which draws attention to this issue, and tries to find support for people who face a need for help in older age without children to provide it. Ageing Well Without Children criticised David Mowat, under-secretary of state for health under Theresa May's government, for arguing that sons and daughters should meet the growing shortfall of eldercare, rather than the state (Asthana, 2017). Jeremy Hunt, health minister in 2015, made a similar call (Woodard, 2015).

---

[2] Ageing Well Without Children, https://www.awwoc.org/

Table 3.1: Trend in number of childless women

Birth decade	Year that oldest reach 80 (if survive)	No. of women	Percentage of cohort who are childless
1920s	2000	42,336	17
1930s	2010	23,178	12
1940s	2020	20,892	11
1950s	2030	35,065	11
1960s	2040	54,706	16
1970s	2050	54,848	19

Source: Office for National Statistics (2024)

Ageing Well Without Children points out that 1.2 million people who are over 65 now have no children, and there will likely be two million of them by 2030.

Disability interacts with the issue of childlessness. The childless include 85 per cent of disabled adults, among them some who are unlikely ever to have partners. They will probably have nobody to help them as they grow older, except their parents or siblings. If they cannot live independently, they often remain in the care of their parents, who may spend very long hours, for decades, looking after a seriously disabled son or daughter.

Even if someone has children, migration means they may not be living within easy reach; disability and work obligations also present barriers to helping parents. Hyacinth's story (Box 3.2) illustrates the difficulties this can cause; friends may or may not fill the gap. Divorce is one factor leading to greater distance of one or other parent from their children. One-fifth of people now in their late 50s live over an hour's journey from their nearest child. Families are also getting smaller; the fewer children someone has, the greater the risk the nearest or only child will live far away (Chan and Ermisch, 2015). Their findings (from 'Understanding Society' data for 2009/10) suggest higher education may increase distance between parents and children. University graduates, a rising proportion of younger people, are more likely to move far from their parents than non-graduates. Only a quarter of UK youth entered university in 2006, but over 38 per cent in 2021

(House of Commons Research, 2024). This factor is also included in the model of Gostoli and Silverman (2019) who found that the 'propensity to care' within different socio-economic groups was differentiated partly by education, which affects internal migration and the probability that someone's children, grandchildren, nieces and nephews will be living in the same town. Fihel et al (2022) found that right across Europe, seniors without children or with only distant children are particularly short of informal help.

Box 3.2: Hyacinth: when children cannot support parents enough

Hyacinth has four children, but feels bereft of family support; two of her daughters live abroad, the other, a two-hour train journey away, visits rarely. Her son lives nearby, but is disabled; she takes him food when she is well enough to travel there. She has several loyal and helpful friends, mainly through her church, but feels it is still not the same as having dependable family to help her with complex paperwork and decisions. (More details in Appendix C)

Rising disability among people under 65

An increasing proportion of younger people have disability support needs. This more than offsets the slight fall in disability among seniors, and is putting a lot of pressure on both local authority services and family members. Disability among working-age adults rose from 15 per cent to 23 per cent during 2010/11 to 2022/3 (House of Commons Research, 2023). More of the working-age adults are needed to look after each other. As the ratio of 'care-needers' to potential 'care-givers' rises, it becomes harder to sustain the volume of informal care.

Long-term health conditions like heart disease, diabetes, arthritis and lung problems are also increasing. They sap the energy of people aged 45–64, the most active age group in providing care for adult family members as well as grandchildren. As future cohorts entering this age group have more long-term health issues, the caring capacity of the working-age population will likely be reduced.

Moreover, the incidence of disability among *future* cohorts of *seniors* will rise as disabled people now of working age get older. The rising prevalence of disability in younger age groups more than offsets the slight decline in disability-related needs among seniors. Thus the ratio of people providing informal care to those who had an 'impairment' fell from one carer per 2.35 'impaired' adults over 16 in 2006/7 to one per 2.61 'impaired' adults in 2018/19. (The FRS defines disability and health problems as 'impairments', a slightly wider definition than the one based on ADLs and IADLs used in the HSE.) Over the whole period 2006/7 to 2018/19, according to the FRS, the ratio of adults without impairments across the UK to disabled adults of *all ages* fell from 3.62 to only 3.0. Impairments included mobility difficulties for over two-fifths of those affected, mental health issues for 44 per cent, and stamina or fatigue problems for over one-third.

Because of family relationships and the relatively high incidence of disability in the most socio-economically deprived groups, the burden of caring is harshly distributed. Many adults who do have a disability, including some who are over 65, actually do care for others, including their partners, their parents if still alive, and their own disabled children (Buckner, 2017). A rising number of parents provide support to disabled adult children, often into the parents' retirement years (Carers UK, 2019, 2022). Jo (see Box 3.3 and Appendix C) is one of them. In 2007/8 only one carer in ten looked after an adult son or daughter, but by 2018/19 this had risen to almost one in five, according to the FRS annual reports. This increase is faster than can be explained by the increasing number of adults under 65 who need support. It suggests that informal care is replacing formal care as council help has shrunk, especially due to the closures of many day centres during the decade of austerity.

Trends in help from non-relatives

Looking at carers for people of all ages, the proportion who look after friends or neighbours, as distinct from relatives, is very small; it remained constant at seven to nine per cent throughout 2006 to 2019, according to the FRS. Among seniors, the proportion helped by non-relatives is considerably larger, as shown in Chapter 2. But the contribution of friends and neighbours appears to have declined substantially over two or three decades. Maher and Green (2002) found from the General Household Survey that 17.2 per cent of carers across Great Britain then looked after friends or neighbours, much more than the FRS shows in later years. However, this difference might arise just from non-comparability of surveys in terms of definitions or design. Two other sources do however show a decline in support from non-kin within a single survey; Hirst (2002, 2005), using the British Household Panel Survey, found that caring by friends and neighbours declined during the 1990s, being replaced by more intensive care from partners and adult children. Similarly, the General Household Survey showed a falling proportion of people over 65 receiving any care from non-relatives between 1985 and 1995 (Pickard, 2002), from a quarter of recipients to just under one-fifth.

The challenge is how to reverse this long-term decline. It is the opposite of what is needed in an era of shrinking and more dispersed families. The childless and those with few or no siblings must look to their friends as the new potential 'family', especially after first their parents and then their partner pass away. But seniors are challenged by friendship networks becoming depleted through death and illness as their peer group ages; intergenerational contacts are especially important to develop sources of support. However, socially close friends of whatever age are not always suitable or available to become a support network; a careful distinction must be made between friendship, support and care (Keating et al, 2003). A large and varied array of personal friendships and acquaintances facilitates instrumental support, but does not guarantee it; this topic is explored further in Chapter 5. *Personal* care, however, is very much a task for household members and professionals.

Employment and pension issues which affect caring

The trade-off between paid work hours and caring hours means that the gradually rising employment rates of older women also pose a threat to informal care provision, as does any rise in the state pension age. Carers were also less likely to be employed (Carmichael et al, 2010). From 2000 to 2022, the employment rate of 50–64-year-old women, the age group most involved in informal care, rose by almost a quarter, from 53.3 per cent to 66.3 per cent.[3]

Over the period 2010 to 2015, successive age cohorts of women had the starting age for their state pension raised in stages from 60 to 65. The pension age for both women and men has since been raised to 66, and further increases are on the horizon. This impacts the capacity of middle-aged women, and more recently of men, to provide informal care. Carrino et al (2020) analysed a sample of 7,102 women aged 55 to 65 across the UK, from the Understanding Society longitudinal survey. Following work and care patterns over the period 2009 to 2017, they estimated that women in this age band are much less likely to provide care for 20 hours or more a week if they have paid work. Those employed 40 hours weekly provided on average only three hours of care per week, but retired women over six hours. However, over 28 per cent of women in the sample provided *some* informal care, whether in employment or not. Thus, raising the retirement age is unlikely to affect the probability of providing *some* care, but likely to reduce the number of hours women provide and especially their availability for intensive care. Carino et al's study also showed that women's working hours fall away only gradually in the six years after pension age. Retired women may continue to depend to some extent on earnings, facing a choice between employment and care.

Carmichael et al (2010) followed individuals of working age moving in and out of caring roles in the longitudinal British Household Panel Survey between 1991 and 2005. They found that people who took up caring roles averaged lower earnings before doing so than those of the same gender who remained non-carers. Caring, especially intensive caring, is more common among lower income groups and in deprived areas (Aldridge and Hughes, 2016). Poorer people are more likely to have relatives

---

[3] Labour Force Survey data, https://www.ons.gov.uk/employmentandlabour market/peopleinwork/employmentandemployeetypes/timeseries/lf2u/lms

in poor health, and to be in poor health themselves, as well as being less able to afford formal care which is no longer free except for the very poorest. Conversely, Carmichael's team found that people with higher hourly pay were less likely to be caring for over 20 hours weekly or reside with the cared-for person. At higher income levels, the preferred choice may be to pay for a relative to have formal care instead (Gostoli and Silverman, 2019).

The substitution debate: would informal care shrink in response to more formal care?

Another threat to the 'supply' of informal care which must be considered is the risk of *unplanned* substitution of formal for informal care, in response to formal care becoming more easily available. What would 'unplanned' mean? Obviously the purpose of expanding subsidised care is, firstly, to meet unmet needs of those receiving insufficient help from informal carers, and especially those who cannot afford to buy care privately. Secondly, it is to help carers who themselves have disabilities or poor health. Thirdly, it is to relieve carers who are doing very long hours. But what if people who have been helping their relatives for only a few hours per week give up, expecting that formal carers will now take their place? And what if a switch from privately purchased homecare to subsidised care exceeds policy makers' expectations, leading to unexpected demand on budgets?

It seems that relatives did take the place of formal care services when they were disrupted by the COVID-19 pandemic, but sometimes under enormous strain. Sons and daughters increased their caring roles during 2011 to 2018 as formal services were cut back. Would informal care fall back again if formal care became more easily available?

Researchers have long been concerned with the question of whether making formal care more easily available, or cheaper, would lead unpaid carers to withdraw. There are some important lessons from what happened in Scotland after FPC was introduced for over-65s in 2002. When the policy was being designed, there were fears of a large increase in demand from people switching out of unpaid care or care they were paying for privately; and there was little data on the latter (Bell et al, 2007a; Holtham, 2018). Several research studies followed to see if the policy did lead to a greater-than-planned substitution of formal care in place of informal care. They form part of a much wider international literature on the 'substitution debate' going back to the 1990s (Chappell and Blandford, 1991; Bonsang, 2009; Zigante et al, 2021). The broad conclusion is that very little shrinkage of informal care occurs when the offer of formal care improves. Nonetheless the Scottish research reveals some interesting issues about unmet need. It also provides complex answers to the question of how informal carers respond when the promised offer of formal care is constrained by underfunding.

Statistics about FPC in Scotland are available only from 2006/7, since after the policy began in 2002 it took some time for reporting systems from local authorities to settle down. From 2006/7 until 2009/10, uptake of FPC rose by almost 15 per cent to about 47,000 clients, but then levelled off (Bell, 2018). Was this because most relevant needs had been met? The answer seems to be almost certainly no; there was an issue of insufficient resources. That may have constrained any shift from informal to formal care. Because of limited local authority budgets, the policy of free assistance with ADLs led to a contraction of *other* forms of formal care such as help with shopping and housework, from around 57,000 recipients in 2006/7 to 49,000 in 2015/16 (Bell, 2018). These 'non-personal' forms of care remain subject to some charges and a means test. Local councils have often increased charges for them to leave sufficient funds for FPC, which they had a statutory obligation to provide. Day centre services also shrank for lack of funding, providing a reason for informal care *not* to fall. Some local authorities over-ran their budgets (Bell et al, 2007a), and 'rationing' of care appeared through lengthening of queues for assessment and referral (Oung, 2020). Perhaps informal carers would have done less had it not been for these developments.

Most local authorities said the new policy was underfunded, even though the Scottish government had recognised the risk of shrinkage of privately purchased care and allowed £10 million to cover its effect on demand. But it was difficult to predict the size of budget needed, since insufficient information was available on private purchases (Holtham, 2018).

Altogether, counting FPC and other homecare for older people – like help with housework – as well as homecare for younger age groups, the number of recipients fell slightly from 2010 onwards (Scottish Government, 2019b), but the average number of hours per client increased slightly, suggesting a rising focus on those with most difficulty (Scottish Government, 2022). Scottish social care spending per head fell slightly in real terms between 2012/13 and 2017/18, to the level reached in Wales (Social Work Scotland, 2020). However, after FPC was extended to all adults in 2019, the number of recipients rose by 13 per cent up to 2022/3 (Scottish Government, 2023). In England, over the same period the number receiving homecare and other 'community care' services rose by only two per cent (NHS Digital, 2024).

FPC in Scotland is defined in a way that helps mainly with ADLs rather than IADLs – it is a right to help with bathing, dressing, eating, using the toilet, and medication. Housework had sometimes been covered by formal services in some areas of Scotland before 2002, but practice varied. There has been some confusion about whether FPC is supposed to help with meal preparation; eventually it was decided that it did not.

One approach to the question of how the Scottish policy affected provision of informal care was to compare trends in Scotland with those in England and Wales (which did not have FPC) over the first two years of the policy (Bell et al, 2007b). Although FRS data showed no difference between the countries, the British Household Panel Survey told a slightly different story when the researchers controlled for other influences on informal caring practices – like age, partnership status, size of household, education and home-ownership. After controlling for the carers' various characteristics, Scotland showed a big reduction in very long hours by informal carers who lived with the cared-for person – mainly partners – compared to what would have been expected without FPC. Those caring for long hours are more likely to be doing personal care, suggesting that the policy helped them to reduce their role, as intended. But there was almost no statistically significant reduction in caring hours of people in Scotland who cared for another household, compared with English data for similar carers. (A slight fall in the probability of women in Scotland caring for another household was significant only at the 10 per cent level.)

Bell et al's model suggests that care is of many different tasks, so that informal carers may respond to free *personal* care either by dropping back or by providing different kinds of care. This would suggest the proportion of the population providing informal care in Scotland may have been sustained because carers moved into meeting other needs which the free formal care services did *not* meet, like housework, paperwork, helping people go out and maybe just keeping them company (Quilter-Pinner and Hochlaf, 2019).

Some substitution of free care services for informal care does seem to have occurred in better-off Scottish households. McNamee (2006), using the Scottish Household Survey, examined how the FPC policy affected provision of informal care in families of different income levels. Before FPC was introduced, there was a tendency for more informal care to be provided in better-off households than in lower-income ones, probably to avoid the expense of self-funded care. Afterwards, the difference in informal care provision between income groups disappeared.

Two other studies showed that people in Scotland were likely to receive *more* informal care because of FPC. Lemmon (2020), using the Scottish Social Care Survey for 2014 to 2016, showed that people receiving FPC had longer hours of informal care than those who did not. This may be because the offer of FPC changed people's choices about whether to enter residential care. Use of long-term residential placements fell since FPC was introduced, possibly because people preferred to stay at home when offered more free help there than before. The FPC policy widened the gap between the costs families faced for residential care, and the cost of care at home, since they still had to pay for the 'hotel costs' of residential placements. The second study, by Karlsberg-Schaffer (2015), used longitudinal data from the British Household Panel Survey, comparing Scotland with the rest of the UK over 2002–10. She found that those who were providing care initially in Scotland continued, and new carers came into the picture mainly offering less than five hours per week. FPC increased the probability of people offering informal care by three to five percentage points, compared to England which did not have FPC. Maybe continuing carers shifted into 'non-personal' care tasks, in line with Bell et al's model. Perhaps also, additional carers came forward to meet these needs when they could be sure that formal carers would take on personal care tasks which are both more demanding and more intimate. They may have been helping relatives or friends who would have gone into residential care before FPC was offered, as McNamee's study suggests. The later trend of informal care in Scotland seems to confirm this. Over the period 2008–19, the percentage of the Scottish population providing some regular unpaid care rose from 11 to 14, according to the Scottish Health Survey.[4] The rise was larger (from 17 to 21 per cent) in the 55–64 age group, the ones most likely to be providing parent-care. This contrasts with the slightly downward trends shown for England and Wales.

Client surveys in Scotland[5] during 2021/2 show an even more rapid increase in informal care than earlier; this was when underfunding had led to reduced satisfaction with FPC services, and COVID-19 led to some homecare packages being reduced or suspended (Fraser of Allender Institute, 2022). Thus, as in England, informal carers stepped into the breach during the pandemic, and it may be too early to say what the long-term trend will be. But what rises may fall; unpaid carers may reduce their support if and when they are confident that formal services are restored.

Overall, studies of the effect of FPC in Scotland find very little substitution of formal care in place of informal care – except possibly for some better-off households who had been struggling to provide enough informal care because with the previous means test their only alternative was self-funding. What did happen was a switch from expensive residential care to receiving more support at home, both paid and unpaid, and possibly a shift of informal care into types of need that had perhaps not previously been sufficiently met. The implementation of FPC did however hit some problems because of underfunding in the early years of the policy – leading, as mentioned earlier, to longer waiting lists

---

[4] https://www.gov.scot/collections/scottish-health-survey/
[5] The annual Scottish Health and Care Experience Survey, https://www.gov.scot/collections/health-and-care-experience-survey/

in some areas, and reduction of other forms of care service like day centres so that local authorities could focus their budgets on FPC. Since the extension of FPC to all adults in 2019, so far these issues have not recurred; 70 to 80 per cent of care assessments are carried out within six weeks, and care is started within the target period of a further six weeks (West, 2024). But local authorities have been squeezed by the spring budget of 2024, and the fear of underfunding of care is reappearing,[6] as it is in England.

The need for new policies to support informal carers

> **Box 3.3: What an intensive carer loses**
>
> Although I managed to return to work part-time, with care worker support at home ... the carers were so unreliable that I eventually took early retirement. ... Unpaid carers are all but abandoned by the state, which takes advantage of them ... the care system in this country is a disgrace for those requiring social care and continuing care. I've lost my career, my retirement I had planned, I've been unable to spend the time I would like with my husband, my other children and my grandchildren, and most important of all, I've lost the wonderful company and smile of my precious daughter. Don't get me wrong, we still enjoy each other's company, but without the laughter and the enthusiastic discussion and banter. (Part of Jo's story; see also Appendix C)

Stress for unpaid carers, especially 'intensive' and/or elderly carers, places in question just how much informal carers can be expected to provide, especially with the very limited financial and other forms of support currently offered by public services. Jo's story shows the intensity of the responsibilities they sometimes carry (see Box 3.3 and Appendix C). Competing demands of paid work and caring, their own health and wellbeing and that of the cared-for person, together with low income and often isolation from activities and people outside the home, present

---

[6] Podcast by the Convention of Scottish Local Authorities, 10 March 2024, https://www.cosla.gov.uk/budget

difficult choices and much distress. Carers are less satisfied with life (Petrie and Kirkup, 2018), feeling a lack of sufficient leisure time if they provide care for more than 10 hours per week. Mental wellbeing and quality of sleep are also affected. The COVID-19 pandemic and the subsequent build-up of waiting lists for hospital admissions, for residential care placements and for assessments to start receiving a care package, has placed unpaid carers under unprecedented strain, according to Association of Directors of Adult Social Services reports (ADASS, 2022b). Carer burnout has frequently led to a breakdown of informal care arrangements (Care Management Matters, 2023). Waiting times for residential placements have also risen by 40 per cent since 2010.

Carer stress and lack of support present an obvious constraint on the sustainability of current levels of informal caring. The HSE provides a bleak picture of support obtained by carers from local authorities or the National Health Service; in 2017 no support was recorded for 56 per cent of carers. Less than one in ten had help from a formal care service. Only one in 20 had advice from their local authority, 3 per cent help or advice from a charity, and only one in 50 had access to respite care (HSE, 2017). Day care, residential respite placements or 'sitter' services, have all declined substantially since 2015/16 due to budget cuts (Nuffield Trust, 2023).

The projections of future care demand mentioned earlier in this chapter estimated that to keep the probability of receiving informal eldercare constant, the amount provided from people other than seniors' partners would need to rise by up to 60 per cent between 2015 and 2035. However, it seems doubtful whether this will happen without some changes in supporting policies. Women who were available to offer informal care in the past are now more likely to be in paid work. They – and men – need time off or more flexible hours for caring for elders, just as they often now request for childcare.

Better carer's leave from their jobs, preferably paid, could help to sustain the capacity for family care. Just as improvements in maternity leave have become an important part of workers' rights in recent decades, leave to care for ageing and/or disabled loved ones needs to improve as well. Employers as well as the state need to support informal carers much more. The UK has poor provision of carer's leave and carer's allowances by international standards. The Carer's Leave Act, which came into force in Britain (except in Northern Ireland) in April 2024, allows people engaged in 'long term care' to have merely one week's leave per year, unpaid. Elfrida's story (Box 3.4) shows how important it can be to have more time off to care for a relative in emergencies.

Box 3.4: Elfrida: when families need carer's leave

Elfrida's daughters, one living abroad, just could not support her enough in four months of crisis. They had used almost all available leave from their jobs after their father died. Shortly afterwards, this lady in her 80s needed a knee operation at a time not of her choosing – while still in the middle of a house move as well as sorting out her husband's complex estate. The two daughters working in London could only visit at weekends, as did one grandson. Most of the time in between, Elfrida had to hobble to her kitchen and bathroom alone. (More of Elfrida's story in Appendix C.)

Box 3.5 shows some examples of far more generous policies from other Organisation for Economic Co-operation and Development countries, albeit often with restrictive conditions about the employee's contract or the health situation of the person they care for (Hamblin et al, 2024).

Several European countries have introduced cash allowances which can be used to pay for user-chosen personal assistants, including close family members, in the hope of sustaining informal care and reducing the cost of formal services (Degavre and Nyssens, 2014). An exemplary policy is in Denmark, where the maximum cash allowance for caring for a relative is 25,138 kroner per month, or around £2,923. This would pay for over 50 hours of care per week at the UK minimum wage. Such an arrangement is offered only where the alternative would be residential care.[7] However, the Danish facility is very little used because formal

---

[7] European Commission, Employment, Social Affairs and Inclusion, Moving and Working in Europe (2023) at https://ec.europa.eu/social/main.jsp?catId=1107&langId=en&intPageId=4491

> **Box 3.5: Examples of carer's leave policies**
>
> There is a legal right to several weeks or months leave in many Organisation for Economic Co-operation and Development countries and even paid leave in some. Good practice examples might be:
>
> - Canada: 55 per cent of salary (up to a ceiling) for up to 26 weeks to care for a relative at significant risk of death within six months; some variation between provinces.
> - France: up to six months paid leave to care for a terminally ill relative.
> - Italy: up to two years over your whole working life to care for sick relatives, on full pay up to a ceiling.
> - Norway: 60 days on full pay to care for a relative or someone 'with close ties'.
> - Sweden: 100 days at 80 per cent of pay to care for someone with a life-threatening illness (OECD, 2020; Hamblin et al, 2024).

homecare is free and easily available. In Germany, cash allowances are an alternative to receiving homecare services in kind; both are options among the benefits of the long-term care insurance system.[8] Germany has five levels of allowance according to need. The cash allowance, or a mix of it with formal care, is by far the most popular arrangement, even though its value per hour of care is only two-fifths of the 'personal budget' rate awarded for formal homecare. This is perhaps because of the availability of underpaid care assistants that households can hire, but also because having just a few hours of formal care for washing and dressing permits the residual 'services in kind' value to be taken as a cash allowance for a family member to do other tasks, enough to pay for over 30 hours care per week at the UK 'living wage'. The danger of providing cash allowances with little oversight from the authorities is that they may result, for example in Germany and Italy, in a 'grey market' of cash-in-hand employment of underpaid people, often migrants and almost always women. This has led the

---

[8] Handbook Germany, 2024, https://handbookgermany.de/en/home-care

German government to offer tax breaks for families who hire care assistants on regular employment contracts (Frericks et al, 2014).

In Germany, informal carers of care allowance recipients are entitled to four weeks' break each year (with care insurance paying the costs of respite care). Their pension and accident insurance contributions are also paid if they are not in full-time paid work and providing 14 or more hours care per week.[9] Rights to regular respite care also exist in Denmark and Finland.

Another possibility to be considered here is how a universal basic income, rather like a child benefit for adults (Miller, 2019), could ease carer stress and help to sustain informal care. This is a popular demand for the reform of income maintenance benefits in many countries, including Scotland, which has considered local experiments to implement it although eventually opting to research a modified Minimum Income Guarantee targeted at lower income groups (IPPR, 2021; Cantillon and O'Toole, 2022). Either scheme would provide every adult with a minimal income, unconditional on employment status or job search behaviour. It would therefore encourage people to take up caring, particularly if such obligations arise sporadically or without notice. It would also enable them to work shorter hours if they needed to make time to care for a relative or friend. To arrange time for caring through easing of the 'work search' obligation in the claimant commitment for Universal Credit requires negotiation with a job coach about whether the claimant meets the criterion of 'regular and substantial caring responsibilities for a severely disabled person'. The fear of being refused benefit if this criterion is considered not to be met may deter people from undertaking care, especially if the need arises suddenly.

Carer's Allowance of £81.90 per week in 2024/5 cannot compensate for lost earnings, being equal to less than one day's pay at the minimum legal wage. It is not available alongside a full state pension and the person cared for must be receiving certain disability-related benefits, with tough and complex eligibility criteria. To claim Carer's Allowance, someone must be caring for at least 35 hours weekly and have net earnings under £151;

---

[9] EuroCarers, the European Association Working for Carers (2024) at https://eurocarers.org/country-profiles/

in Scotland there is an extra supplement of £288.60 paid twice a year. Current rules present a benefits trap; a carer who breaches the earnings limit loses the whole sum.

Disabled seniors in Great Britain who need care can claim Attendance Allowance, currently £72.65 or the higher rate of £108.55 if 24-hour supervision is needed. They can use this to pay a relative if they want. But only in exceptional circumstances can co-resident relatives be paid with a 'personal budget' provided by the local authority. This would be a welcome change, bringing UK policy on this point into line with Germany and Denmark.

Informal carers badly need recognition and encouragement. They also provide care with virtually no overhead costs, so paying them rather than a care agency could make public money go further. Much higher remuneration for intensive carers is worthy of further research, to see if it could incentivise informal care and ease carer poverty and stress. End Social Care Disgrace, a lobbying organisation for carers, has recently discussed a possible demand for a wage-replacement income for intensive carers, permitting them to claim the national living wage for caring hours. The cost of this is considered in Chapter 4.

Conclusion

This chapter has described the challenges of expanding care sufficiently to cope with the needs of an ageing society. To meet these needs firstly requires a major expansion of subsidised *formal* care. There is considerable unmet need for help with ADLs, as shown in Chapter 2. If relatives have reached their limits or are in short supply, as with childless singles, formal care is vital to meet these needs. This kind of intimate personal care can only be done by close kin or professional services, which many people cannot afford. Even if the 'propensity to care (unpaid)' can be sustained, demographic and cost pressures alone indicate a huge escalation of care costs over coming years. Based on the modelling work of the Personal Social Services Research Unit team described in this chapter, the Health Foundation (2023) estimated that the care budget would need to rise by almost 47 per cent between 2023/4 and 2032/3 alone. This challenge is further examined in Chapter 4.

Secondly, there is a need to sustain and encourage informal care, and reduce conflicts between paid work and caring, by providing informal carers with much greater support services and financial help. There are several ways to do this which seem achievable in other European countries, such as longer paid carer's leave from employment and better cash allowances for full-time carers.

Carer's Allowance needs drastic reform and should be made into a proper income for work done, rather than carrying conditions about maximum earnings from paid work. While special benefits need to be preserved and increased for full-time carers and those they look after, a basic income would help to free other people for caring responsibilities, by helping them to work shorter hours or to take unpaid leave if called on to provide care in emergencies.

The several threats to sustaining the 'propensity to care' suggest a need to provide more community support both to care-needers and family carers. Ways of doing this, through various forms of mutual aid and through widening personal support networks, are discussed in Chapters 5 and 6. This is important to keep the formal care budget from falling short of needs, especially in the short term; reform of the present care system may take several years. But informal care from beyond close family does not, and cannot, *replace* the core task of state services; that is, personal care, which occupies the greatest part of what formal services currently do. Rather, community solidarity can contribute to meeting a wider range of needs in the hope of delaying and reducing individuals' need for formal care. Chapters 5 and 6 will examine how this might be done, while not detracting from the need to secure sufficient growth of formal services.

4

Who pays? How much care could be free, what kinds and for whom?

Introduction

The demand for free personal care, modelled on the Scottish policy, has become popular further south in recent years. As noted in Chapter 1, many organisations want a national social care service, to be free at the point of use, and funded nationally like the NHS, rather than locally. People are asking, if Scotland can make care free, why not England? It would cost much more than the very limited care reforms once planned for autumn 2025, then abandoned in the tight fiscal regime of July 2024. But as this chapter will show, the amounts of money required to pay care workers adequately and meet unmet needs are substantially larger than the cost of abolishing user charges. Care reform requires bold steps to raise more public funds. The clamour of so many organisations for free social care is a popular and worthy long-term objective which has also been adopted by the Welsh government for the long term (Welsh Government, 2023). However, one needs to be realistic about what can be achieved quickly, and to consider how to prioritise different care reforms.

Any increase in care subsidies cannot depend on the regressive, geographically uneven and inadequate yields of council tax. The most urgent requirement, even before reducing charges, is a major injection of funds from national sources to avoid further cuts. In early 2024, several English councils were on the verge of bankruptcy, and social services directors worried about how they would meet even current costs (Samuel, 2024). Beyond keeping existing services going, should the priority be reducing or abolishing charges for existing clients, or improving quality of care, meeting unmet needs or easing the load on unpaid carers? There are complex choices about what kinds of care should be subsidised and for whom.

The cost estimates here cover all adults. Although this text focuses on seniors, there is no reason to prioritise them over younger disabled adults, who show the most rapid growth in demand for formal care, and often need much more support than seniors. The most severely impaired, their parents and partners may face several decades of *unpaid* caring, with poverty due to difficulties of maintaining paid work and often extra costs of transport or heating.

Any proposal for 'free care' needs to define what that includes. At present, just a small corner of the service is free under means-tested arrangements. How much *more* should be free, what kinds of care and for whom? Given the vast scale of unpaid care described in Chapter 2, formal services could not possibly replace it all.

The Scottish model of a universal free service, based on assessment of clinical need, has been inspirational, despite some early difficulties noted in Chapter 3. But it is just for 'personal care'; most people still pay for the means-tested 'board and lodging' costs of residential care. Free personal care (FPC) is quite narrowly defined; help with 'activities of daily living' like bathing, dressing, getting around indoors and toilet needs, but not cleaning, mobility support, meal preparation, day services or home adaptations. Up to two-thirds of people receiving home care in Scotland before the FPC policy was introduced had needs it didn't meet, and for which they still pay[1] – including general supervision of people with dementia, support to attend social activities, or help with laundry.

Another major challenge is to raise care workers' wages to a level adequate for recruitment and retention of the workforce. There are key trade-offs between paying care workers more, helping

---

[1] Nuffield Trust blog, 3 October 2019, https://www.nuffieldtrust.org.uk/news-item/what-might-labour-s-free-personal-care-pledge-actually-mean

more people and reducing user charges. To some extent, this can be balanced by several ways to reduce the cost of care through some possible changes in forms of provision, which frequently offer quality improvements too. These are considered later in this chapter; helping more people avoid costly and unpopular residential care, expanding not-for-profit care provision, more flexible homecare packages, and proper pay for informal carers.

Appendix A provides details of the cost estimates and suggests possible sources of revenue for expanding the care budget. Sadly, the estimates discussed here exclude Wales and Northern Ireland. The main sources about demand for care and its costs, the Association of Directors of Adult Social Services returns, the HSE and the English Longitudinal Study of Ageing (ELSA) are all for England only.

Choices about charging: limited free care for all, or a wider range of services with some charges?

Should subsidies be focused on those with greatest clinical need or financial need? Should they be spread across a wider range of services? Inaffordability of care is a serious issue; over 60,000 people were pursued for care charge debts in 2020/1.[2] Some don't apply for council care because of the likely co-payment. But others are not even offered the choice because councils lack capacity, with long waits even for assessment.

The Fabian Society (Harrop and Cooper, 2023) opposes the Scottish focus on *personal* care, questioning whether this is the most important range of services for everyone. But against spreading the subsidy over a wider range of services, prioritising *personal* care can be defended in two ways. It is the range of tasks which is most difficult for any informal carer but a partner, son or daughter to do; and the greatest care deficit is felt by those without close relatives to help. Secondly, if the personal care entitlement is offered as a 'personal budget', recipients could actually spend it as they wish; if they hire a personal assistant, what tasks she or he covers can be negotiated between them.

---

[2] BBC News, 22 February 2023, https://www.bbc.co.uk/news/uk-64668729

The current English system focuses subsidy on those with lowest incomes, although the means test thresholds have been unchanged for over a decade. The 'lifetime cost cap', proposed in 2023 in England (Department of Health and Social Care et al, 2022), but abandoned in July 2024, was criticised for favouring those with substantial assets to lose when paying for residential care (Sturrock and Tallack, 2022). The alternative Welsh approach has been to place a cap on weekly homecare charges, currently at £120, while planning eventually to make homecare free.[3] This weekly cap focuses homecare subsidy on those with need for the longest hours of service. Only if someone needs care for over 13 years would they be better off with the now-shelved proposal to cap lifetime costs at £86,000. However, the case for a lifetime cap, which could be made more progressive than the abandoned proposal of 2023–4, is defended by the Health Foundation (2024), since FPC alone would still leave huge 'hotel' costs to cover for someone who needs residential care for many years.

The four countries of the UK differ about the level of assets above which someone must pay for all their care home fees; it is £23,250 in both England and Northern Ireland, £32,750 in Scotland and £50,000 in Wales (House of Commons Library, 2022). In Scotland, anyone with over £32,750 pays the full *accommodation costs* of residential care, although personal and nursing care is free.

Although means testing is unpopular, just abolishing all charges without changing the tax system would give most gains to higher-income clients, without improving the size or quality of care packages. Should better-off people still pay something? Should some charges be retained to improve service quality? The Fabian Society considers several other options:

- Making all services free, regardless of income, to those with the greatest medical need or disabled from an early age. This would help not only the most needy clients but their hard-pressed informal carers.

---

[3] https://socialcare.today/2024/02/28/welsh-government-announces-20-rise-in-adult-care-charge-cap/

- Reforming the means test, with higher thresholds for self-funding to begin. (Part of the English charging reform planned for autumn 2025, but abandoned in July 2024,[4] took this option.)
- Making services partially free to all those with support needs. This could involve a Welsh-style weekly cap on care costs, with a percentage co-payment for services up to the level of the cap.

Whatever form of subsidy is chosen, offering it as a personal budget is important, so that users can change or vary the services they use. Personal budgets need to be index-linked to ensure they are not eroded as service costs rise. Any means test, if retained, also needs to be index-linked. But means-testing may be seen as a tax on disability, which could be more fairly replaced by more tax on high incomes and wealth.

Care Act guidance is ambiguous about how much can be expected of family carers. In practice, as shown in Chapter 2, there is considerable reliance on partners, and single people receive rather more formal services. Budget projections need different scenarios about how much informal carers can be expected to do. This in turn depends on the availability of respite and day care, carer's leave, and the scale of carer's allowances.

Two London local authorities have pioneered free social care. Tower Hamlets plans to abolish charges for homecare from April 2025.[5] Hammersmith and Fulham already abolished homecare charges in 2015. Then there were 313 people paying some contribution, out of 1,266 who received homecare.[6] There was no apparent rush to take free council care instead of private purchases of homecare. By 2020 the number receiving homecare had risen only to 1,336, perhaps helped by increased support services to informal carers. Average weekly hours provided per client (29.9

---

[4] BBC, 30 July 2024, https://www.bbc.co.uk/news/articles/c3g9m7p199no
[5] 'Real' (a voluntary group) blog, 8 March 2023, https://www.real.org.uk/news/statement-on-abolishing-social-care-charging-in-tower-hamlets/; and personal communication from the LB Tower Hamlets press office indicates that implementation will now be in April 2025.
[6] Hammersmith and Fulham Council press release, 4 December 2014, https://www.lbhf.gov.uk/news/2014/12/tax-disability-be-abolished

hours) were almost double the 2020 London average (15.1 hours).[7] Losing around £340,000 in charges income was made affordable by savings on council publications budgets, including scrapping the magazine previously sent to every household. A means test remains for residential care.

Unmet need and the cost of meeting it

Age UK (2023b) estimated that around 1.4 million people over 65 have some unmet needs for care in 2023, based on their analysis of ELSA. Taking the average for all those receiving formal homecare in ELSA data of 2018/19, around 11.5 hours per week, these 1.4 million people, if they *all* depended on that amount of formal care, would need 16.1 million hours of care between them per week. That would be many times the capacity of the care system; in the first three months of 2022, local authorities delivered only 1.1 million hours per week. Most people depend on informal care, as shown in Chapter 2. Even in Scotland, where personal care is free, the number of unpaid carers is over ten times the number of people receiving homecare (Scottish Government Health and Social Care, 2021).

It is difficult to translate Age UK's finding into an estimate of need for formal services. Not everyone assessed as *needing* formal care actually *wants* it; there are issues of privacy and loss of independence. Although less than 13 per cent of seniors with activities of daily living (ADL) difficulties in the HSE sample for 2018 used homecare or cleaners, some of the remaining 87 per cent thought they could manage without help. Others, and their relatives, may be content to rely on family care alone. Those without formal care probably need fewer weekly hours than current recipients, since local authorities focus on higher-need cases.

However, many people have unmet needs while awaiting assessment; the queue has become much longer in recent years.

---

[7] Hammersmith and Fulham Council (2020) *Homecare Needs Assessment 2020–21*. https://democracy.lbhf.gov.uk/documents/s122363/BACKGROUND%2520DOC%2520-Homecare%2520Needs%2520Assessment%2520Report%25202020-21.pdf

Waiting lists had over 225,000 people across England in March 2023, over a quarter of them having waited longer than six months (Institute for Government, 2023). By March 2024, 470,476 people were waiting for either assessment, review or for care to actually *begin* (Public Accounts Committee, 2024). After assessment, only a small fraction of those making requests actually receive homecare or a residential placement. Many are referred to other forms of support – such as alarm systems, home adaptations, voluntary sector support or universal services like benefits advice. This may be all they need, or a 'second best' induced by shortage of funding or staff. Over a quarter of those making requests receive no services, because their needs are not considered serious enough, or their council is short of capacity, or they decline services on finding they need to pay (Nuffield Trust, 2023).

One way to allow for currently unmet need is to estimate the cost of restoring the level of formal care provision that existed before the 'decade of austerity'. Needs assessments then were more generous. Since 2014, councils are thought to have exercised 'subjective eligibility rationing' because of the shortage of funds (Samuel, 2023). So fewer people received any services. By 2018/19, seniors' care packages averaged ten hours per week, compared to 12 hours in 2009/10 (Bedford and Button, 2022). In 2010, many more people would have been eligible for free care than can qualify now, since the savings thresholds of the means test have been unchanged since 2010/11. The Health Foundation (Alderwick et al, 2019) estimated at £12.5 billion the extra cost of restoring the scope and standards of care to 2010/11 levels, including upgrading carers' pay – implying the budget really needed to be two-thirds more than it was.

Estimating the cost of care with varying assumptions about wage costs and scope of services

This section attempts to estimate the cost of a universal care service if we include better pay for care workers, and extend the service to meet unmet need. It is loosely based on the work of the New Economics Foundation with the Women's Budget Group, referred to in what follows as NEF/WBG for short (Bedford and Button, 2022). They used projections of the ongoing rise in demand for care by the CPEC research unit (formerly the Personal Social Services Research Unit) at the London School of Economics and Political Science, which also underly the Health Foundation's research. NEF/WBG made use of another Health Foundation paper (Rocks et al, 2021), which suggested increasing total care hours by one-tenth to serve more people and/or more hours per client, and raising the hourly rate paid by councils to care providers by 18 per cent. In considering what level of hourly fees providers need, Health Foundation researchers took the yardstick of the billing rate then recommended by the UK Home Care Association (UKHCA). This was based on paying care workers the National Living Wage (NLW), and included enough for travel time between clients. But is the NLW enough?

The NEF/WBG go somewhat further in the extent to which they accommodate both unmet need and better care workers' pay. The author's adaptation and updating of their estimates is shown in Appendix A.

Alternative definitions of need and different scenarios about who should receive formal care

The NEF/WBG calculated the total care budget needed without any user charges, to service all those in need of care according to definitions described shortly. These care-needers include those without any formal care, those who pay their local authority for all or part of their service, and others who buy their own care from private sources.

The NEF/WBG methodology has alternative scenarios about who is considered in need of formal care. They calculated demand at two levels of need, based on data from the HSE for over-65s, and from the Family Resources Survey for younger adults:

- 'LA needs' is the level of eligibility used by local authorities under the definitions of the Care Act 2014 for 'severe needs'; for seniors, this is taken to be people who can't manage two or more ADLs alone without difficulty. For under 65s, the NEF/WBG assumed that 26 per cent of those identified as 'severely disabled' in the Family Resources Survey meet 'LA needs' criteria, each needing 21 hours care per week.

- 'Wider needs' included other seniors who need long-term help, because of a health condition and difficulties with at least one ADL, or at least two instrumental activities of daily living or mobility issues. For under-65s, the remaining quarter of 'severely disabled' people are thought to require two hours of care per week.

Their estimates show four alternative levels of homecare take-up for seniors with 'LA needs':

- current use of formal homecare (19 per cent of those with severe needs);
- take-up if FPC was offered (29 per cent);
- a higher use of formal services to relieve informal carers who do over 19 hours weekly (68 per cent);
- 100 per cent, replacing all informal care (shown by NEF/WBG for comparison, this would be horrendously expensive).

The take-up rate for FPC is based on Scottish experience. Offering *free* personal care to seniors would, NEF/WBG thought, induce uptake of formal *homecare* use by 29 per cent of clients with 'LA needs', or 49 per cent of available hours. Apparently not all private purchasers take up free care if it is offered, maybe to maintain continuity or superior quality. But the ones who need more hours are more likely to take it up, so the take-up is higher when measured in hours. However, switching from private purchases to free care is inherently unpredictable, as the Scottish government found in 2002 (Holtham, 2018).

The need for higher pay for care workers

One major determinant of costs is the need for much higher pay for care sector workers. Although the NLW has risen rapidly in recent years, even their employers are now calling for much more.

Some detail on care workers' pay is needed to understand how large a pay rise may be needed. A study of residential care workers found that dire poverty entails food insecurity for at least one in ten of their families (Allen, 2022). While Hammersmith and

Fulham require all homecare agencies they use to pay the Real Living Wage, many local authorities do not. Cash-strapped local authorities offer very low rates to care agencies, who pass on this pressure to their staff. According to the union UNISON, three-quarters of care workers are not paid for travel time,[8] although it takes up to one-fifth of their working hours. Over two-fifths of homecare workers have zero-hours contracts, making their income potentially erratic and insecure (Skills for Care, 2023). The impact goes beyond their poverty; the care sector has 130,000 unfilled vacancies in 2024. Pay rises focused on meeting the legal minimum have narrowed differentials for senior staff, leading to insufficient opportunity for salary progression (Dayan, 2023). This impacts staff retention; 29 per cent of the workforce leave their jobs every year.[9]

Labour costs are over 70 per cent of the care budget, so the funds needed are hugely influenced by wage rates. The NLW, currently £11.44 per hour in 2024/5, has not kept pace with living costs. The Living Wage Foundation invites employers to pledge a higher rate; a 'Real Living Wage' of £13.15 in London and £12 elsewhere in the UK.[10] Strikes of NHS staff for higher pay in 2023–4, the high minimum earnings threshold for migrant workers to obtain a work visa, and difficulty recruiting to the care sector, all suggest that a much higher hourly pay rate is needed. It has often been argued that expanding subsidised care creates jobs; but the current problem seems to be that vacant care jobs are hard to fill.

The care home providers' association, Care England, suggested that £15 per hour was needed in 2023 to maintain a sufficient differential over competing jobs. This £15 wage is fed into the overall estimate of care costs developed here. It is also the

---

[8] UNISON, https://www.unison.org.uk/news/2023/06/majority-of-home care-staff-are-unpaid-for-travel-between-visits-says-unison/
[9] UK Home Care Association, https://www.homecareassociation.org.uk/resource/workforce-trends-in-the-homecare-sector-a-deep-dive-into-turnover-rates.html
[10] Living Wage Foundation, https://www.livingwage.org.uk/news/living-wage-foundation-responds-announcement-governments-national-living-wage-rise-april-2024

minimum homecare wage recommended by the UKHCA for 2024 (Booth, 2023), but below the £15.21 recommended by the Scottish Women's Budget Group (2023).

Could care agencies absorb a major pay rise without charging councils more? In recent years care industry sources, the National Audit Office (2021) and the UKHCA (2023) have all said that billing rates were too low for viability. Following the rise of almost one-tenth in the NLW in 2023, over two-fifths of agencies closed some branches or withdrew from council contracts they considered unprofitable. Profit margins are frequently less than 5 per cent. Many companies make an overall loss despite charging higher rates to self-funders. Local authorities can influence carers' wages through the contract conditions they use for providers, but only if they pay enough. The UKHCA (2023) estimated that to pay the hourly National Living Wage of £11.44 in 2024, agencies would need at least £28.53 per hour of care – more than what many local authorities paid.

A major goal of care reform, therefore, must be to find ways to pay care workers more while charging clients less. This clearly requires a huge input of extra national funding to avoid a cruel choice between exploiting care workers and the amount or quality of services offered. There is an equity issue here between clients and workers; although some people are reduced to poverty by care charges, or see their children's chance of home-ownership eroded as family savings trickle away, some self-funders and their families may be considerably better off than their paid carers. However, people with high incomes or assets but no need for care are better off still, which argues for taxation to fund care rather than charges.

How different wage scenarios affect funding requirements

The NEF/WBG considered three different options for average care workers' pay per hour. Each included pension contributions, sick and holiday pay as extra costs:

1. the very low actual wage level of 2019/20, around £8.87;
2. a 'Real Living Wage' option of £10 (50p more than the Real Living Wage of 2019/20);

3. a 'Nordic' option of £13.19, so-called because it parallels the much higher wages for carers found in Denmark, Norway and Sweden. This implied a pay rise of 49 per cent on UK levels of 2019/20, plus substantial investment in training. Later, writing about Scotland, the same researchers updated the level to £15.21 for 2023. (Scottish Women's Budget Group, 2023)

NEF/WBG's estimates included £4.5 billion for other costs such as administration and assessment, 'hotel costs' of residential and nursing care, and an annual visit from a nurse for everyone over 75. Although requiring 8,420 nurses for England, this has been found to be a valuable preventive service in Denmark, helping to anticipate needs and reduce the requirement for care services. Allowing for inflation, the £4.5 billion might now be £5 billion.

The NEF/WBG estimated that the total gross care budget just to meet formal care take-up by people with 'LA needs' (two or more ADL difficulties plus a low wellbeing score) needed to be at least £31 billion in 2021/2 at the then *current* wage levels, covering both homecare and the costs of care in residential/nursing care. This figure implied an extra £12 billion over actual public net spending in 2021/2, all due to meeting unmet 'LA needs', before raising wages or reducing charges. If care workers had a slightly higher wage, averaging £10 per hour, the budget rose in the NEF/WBG calculations to £39.9 billion at 2021/22 prices. The NEF/WBG's 'Nordic option', with a £13.19 wage, led to an estimate of £48.6 billion for 2021/2. The next section examines what happens with even higher wages, as now seems necessary.

The NEF/WBG's preferred scenario has a higher take-up by seniors, in which informal help of over 19 hours weekly would be replaced by formal care. They estimate that offering this to relieve intensive family carers would mean 68 per cent of seniors with 'severe' needs receiving formal care. Relieving informal carers in this way adds 21 per cent to the budget compared with just scrapping charges.

The future cost of adult care at adequate wage and billing rates

NEF/WBG estimated that 1.7 million full-time equivalent homecare workers were needed for the 'LA care needs' of the population in 2019/20. But there were only 1.2 million full-time equivalent care workers in 2024,[11] showing how care reform requires much investment in training and recruitment of staff. Like the NEF/WBG, the Institute for Public Policy Research (IPPR; Quilter-Pinner and Hochlaf, 2019) pointed out that many thousands of extra staff would be needed, underlining the need for more attractive pay. Both time and funding needed to recruit and train staff must be considered in any future plan.

The UKHCA's highest recommended hourly billing rate in 2024 is £34.30, based on the actual hourly wage for experienced workers in outer London on NHS pay rate band 3, which is £14.65 (UKHCA, 2023). Adding 35p to provide a £15 wage would mean a billing rate of £34.69.

Assuming, like NEF/WBG, that 29 per cent of over-65s with 'LA need' would actually take up free homecare if offered (or 49 per cent of the hours estimated to be needed), the cost across England in 2024/5 at a £15 wage would be £32.35 billion, according to the calculations in Appendix A, Table A2. For residential and nursing homes, where everyone needs formal care, a £15 wage implies that the actual care element would cost around £15.4 billion per year, as shown in Appendix A, Table A3. Residents would additionally pay means-tested 'hotel costs', even if the care element was free.

Thus, even just for severe needs, homecare and the care element of residential and nursing-home care, at a £15 carers' wage, would cost £47.75 billion. Adding assessment, administration, preventive nurse visits for everyone reaching age 75, and 'hotel costs' of residential care for those who currently get subsidies would mean an extra £5 billion, based on updating NEF/WBG estimates; so altogether £52.75 billion. Still more is needed for home adaptations, day and respite services, plus advice, training and financial support for informal carers.

There would be some offsetting savings. Some of any extra spending on care returns to the state as additional income tax yield (although not if the newly recruited staff were already employed at similar wages elsewhere in the UK). Additionally, meeting

---

[11] King's Fund, https://www.kingsfund.org.uk/insight-and-analysis/data-and-charts/key-facts-figures-adult-social-care

previously *unmet* care needs would save the NHS money, and free some informal carers to work in paid jobs (and pay more taxes). In Scotland, FPC also reduced the need for expensive residential care.

However, if care workers are to be paid anything approaching £15 per hour, it seems that care on an adequate scale, even for all with the 'LA need' or severe needs level, requires tapping several of the extra revenue sources listed in Appendix A, Table A1 – basically taxes on upper income groups. The required budget also needs to be reduced without squeezing providers and care workers. The main way to do this is through prevention, reducing *demand* by keeping healthier – the topic of Chapter 7. Additionally, some *supply-side changes* suggested later in this chapter would help reduce unit costs.

What would it cost to make care free?

Retaining charges, with some clients priced out, would probably save less than £7 billion out of these figures (adding charging income and removing the extra demand induced by making care free). Thus the vast bulk of the cost increase is due to meeting currently unmet need, and raising care workers' pay.

Several estimates have been made for the cost of making all 'personal care' free. Taking Hammersmith and Fulham as an example, a minimum estimate of what is required for free care throughout England would be simply abolishing user charges for care currently arranged by local authorities. These user charges amounted to £3.2 billion[12] in 2020/1, for all adults. However, this measure would not tackle unmet need, nor the inadequacy of care workers' pay.

Looking at other estimates of cost for free care *just for seniors*, Bell (2018) estimated local authorities would need an extra £3.8 billion annually (or around £4.5 billion in 2022/3 prices) for introducing FPC for seniors in England; more than for

---

[12] ASC-FR Collection 2020/21, NHS Digital (Adult Social Care and Finance Reports), https://digital.nhs.uk/data-and-information/publications/statistical/adult-social-care-activity-and-finance-report/2019-20

just abolishing charges, because it includes some allowance for expanding the number of recipients. The IPPR (Quilter-Pinner and Hochlaf, 2019) arrived at similar conclusions. By January 2024, the Health Foundation estimated that FPC for over-65s, based on expanding a free service to all self-funders arranging care through local authorities plus increased demand induced by abolishing charge, would cost £6 billion, rising to £7 billion in 2035/6 (Alderwick et al, 2024). The cost of making care free for all adults after expanding the scope of the service to cover unmet need was estimated at around £5.3 billion in 2022/3 in an earlier paper; this is the difference between the 'free' and 'not free' scenarios in the Technical Annex of Health Foundation (2023). NEF/WBG make it £5 billion with a £10 hourly carer's wage; if carers get £15 per hour it could rise to £7 billion now rather than in the 2030s. For comparison, the Health Foundation estimated that the government's now-abandoned plan for a lifetime cap would have cost £0.5 billion in 2026/7, rising to £3.5 billion in 2035/6.

Help for unpaid carers and its impact on the care budget

A different scenario in the NEF/WBG paper calculates the cost of offering formal services to reduce long hours by family carers. Free formal homecare for everyone with the 'LA need' level *plus* all receiving over 19 hours of informal care raises the budget requirement by almost a quarter. Perhaps this could be partly met by paying informal carers, which cuts out organisational overheads of formal provision. As suggested in Chapter 3, Carer's Allowance could be turned into an income for work done, with no restrictions on other earnings. A campaigning group, End Social Care Disgrace, has considered calling for at least the National Living Wage to be paid to full-time informal carers. To pay 1.36 million current claimants of Carer's Allowance for 35 hours at the national minimum wage would cost over £28 billion. A compromise might be £16.2 billion to pay them just for 20 hours. Probably more people would then claim, adding further to the cost. If adopted as a long-term target, it would need to be implemented in stages over several years. This could be offset against the current cost of Carer's

Allowance (£3.8 billion)[13] and possibly of Attendance Allowance (£6.7 billion).[14]

Paying an informal carer would often be cheaper than the cost of residential care. To illustrate the potential saving, paying a family carer even as much as £15 per hour for 35 hours per week would cost £525, compared to residential care for seniors at £800 to £1,000 or more. The Danish arrangement mentioned in Chapter 3 is an example of how good allowances for family carers may provide an alternative to residential care.

An additional possibility would be the use of personal budgets to pay close relatives, as suggested in Chapter 3 (this could either add to the 20 hours mentioned earlier or partly replace it). A household member cannot generally be paid as a 'personal assistant' under personal budget arrangements, although some exceptions are allowed. Many informal carers are desperate for additional formal care; they need more time, which cannot be replaced by money. But an unemployed or retired household member might welcome permission to be paid as a personal assistant.

The IPPR (Quilter-Pinner and Hochlaf, 2019) suggest repurposing Attendance Allowance to provide a personal budget for people with moderate care needs, thus extending the scope of free care and offering scope to pay informal carers to do it. This could bring up to £7 billion into the available funding, and may be worth further research.

Basic income schemes would be another way to support informal carers. Researchers have produced many costed proposals for a universal basic income (UBI) (Miller, 2019). They argue that UBI would help people make time away from paid work for unpaid care, although disability advocacy groups such as Disabled People Against Cuts (DPAC, 2019) fear that UBI might compete for funding with specific disability-related benefits.

---

[13] Statistica, 12 July 2024, https://www.health.org.uk/sites/default/files/2023-09/ASC%2520Funding%2520Pressures%2520Model%25202023%2520update%2520-%2520TECHNICAL%2520ANNEX.pdf

[14] Statistica, 20 August 2024, https://www.statista.com/statistics/284422/uk-attendance-allowance-expenditure/

Supply-side measures to reduce the unit costs of care

The care budget clearly needs to rise, not fall. So far, this chapter has highlighted the need for a vast increase to meet current and future needs. But there are several ways which might help to make a given national budget go further and improve quality. One is more commissioning of non-profit providers. Another is shifting away from residential care. Chapter 7, as mentioned earlier, addresses a third: prevention and early help.

Cutting costs but not wages: homecare

How could homecare costs be reduced while offering care workers an adequate wage? Service users may wonder why care agencies' billing rates approach 2.5 times the worker's hourly pay. But average profit margins are actually only around 5 per cent, according to the UKHCA (2023). The UKHCA sets out typical costs per hour of care: back-office staff and managers £3.36; non-labour office costs £2.63; staff recruitment £0.36; insurance, regulatory costs and training £1.18. When fully compensated, as it should be, travel time averages £2.70 per hour spent with clients, and mileage expenses £1.89.

Micro-enterprise

A share of these costs, though not all, could be avoided by self-employed workers, particularly with very local clients. Community Catalysts, a social enterprise development organisation,[15] has helped several local authorities develop 'micro-enterprises' to deliver homecare and support with many tasks, including some that formal care services rarely offer; handyperson jobs, help with going out, cleaning, de-cluttering, gardening, managing medical appointments and paperwork, day support and respite care, advice and advocacy. Much of their work is with younger disabled adults who need more of these tasks and less personal care than seniors, but some offer personal care too. Micro-enterprises are small teams of up to ten people, generally working as self-employed

---

[15] Community Catalysts organisational website, www.communitycatalysts.co.uk

partners, but serving multiple clients. They usually work from home, serve very local clients, and avoid the substantial overheads of care agencies, usually charging lower hourly rates (Needham et al, 2017).

In Somerset, Community Catalysts partnered with the County Council to launch a micro-enterprise programme in 2015. Five years later there were over 450 enterprises (Bedford and Phagoora, 2020); by January 2024, 1,215 served almost 6,000 clients, providing 30,000 hours of support per week and saving the council over £900,000 per year.[16] Similar Community Catalyst initiatives have been set up in the West Midlands, Bedfordshire, Suffolk, Westminster and Thurrock.[17]

Micro-enterprises have many advantages compared to larger providers (Needham et al, 2014, 2017). Autonomous self-employed workers can 'co-produce' their service flexibly with the client, responding to changing needs about what to do and preferred hours of visits. Compared to many agencies, they provide greater continuity with little staff turnover, getting to know their clients and providing a more personalised and client-controlled kind of care. Micro-enterprises work well with family and friends of the client, and some have their own volunteers.

The conditions for micro-enterprises to advertise on council websites, and be chosen by clients with their personal budgets, can be designed to drive up quality. An example is provided by Somerset County Council.[18] Their document, *Doing it Right: Quality Standards*, covers public liability insurance, safeguarding issues, Disclosure and Barring Service checks, complaints procedure, contractual arrangements with clients and compliance with Care Quality Commission regulations. Some

---

[16] Somerset County Council, https://www.somerset.gov.uk/care-and-support- for-adults/somerset-micro-enterprise-project/
[17] Association for Public Excellence blog, 2021, https://www.apse.org.uk/index.cfm/apse/news/articles/2021/thurrock-micro-enterprises-ordinary-people-doing-extraordinary-things/#
[18] 'Doing it Right' Quality Standards, https://somersetcc.sharepoint.com/sites/SCCPublic/Social%20Care/Forms/AllItems.aspx?id=%2Fsites%2FSCC Public%2FSocial%20Care%2FThe%20Doing%20It%20Right%20 Quality%20 Standards%2Epdf; Central Bedfordshire Council, (nd).

micro-enterprises are not Care Quality Commission registered, but are required to avoid activities that would demand registration.

Micro-enterprises have some difficulties. Councils prefer to commission services through large-scale block contracts, and may not refer enough clients to a micro-enterprise for it to operate at sufficient scale to be sustainable; getting clients then depends a lot on personal contacts. Somerset groups micro-enterprises into local area networks, which offer opportunities for mutual support and collaboration (Bedford and Phagoora, 2020). This may also help to offer staff rotation and holiday cover, and more choices for clients. Anchor organisations in the community can also offer channels for client referrals and for recruitment of volunteers.

In Somerset, the popularity of micro-enterprises has encouraged increased take-up of personal budgets, which clients need to commission their own services. But in many areas clients have been slow to move to personal budgets, and there may be bureaucratic delays in setting them up.

Micro-enterprises frequently attract people with lengthy experience in the care sector; two-thirds of those in Somerset and Thurrock are over 50 (Bedford and Phagoora, 2020). Although Community Catalysts are careful not to market their schemes for registration and training to existing care workers, many do want to set up on their own. However, micro-enterprises themselves may not have resources to train new, younger workers. This may need local authority investment; for example, Cambridge County Council has offered all care workers access to free training through the Care Professional Academy. Community Catalysts advises new micro-enterprises on locally available training, and with the funding they receive from local authorities, provides various short courses online.

Care cooperatives

The Equal Care Coop, founded in Calderdale, Yorkshire in 2018, is a multi-stakeholder cooperative and registered homecare provider. Its governance model promotes inclusive decision-making and distributed authority and uses its own tech platform to facilitate community co-production of care through local 'circles' and 'teams'. Circle members, including care workers and local community volunteers, collaborate to recruit and match care workers with those seeking support and build self-managing teams. Teams are owned by the person receiving care and support; they can comprise friends, family members, volunteers and Equal Care's vetted care workers. Shared ownership and peer-governance means all stakeholders, giving or receiving paid or unpaid care, participate in strategic decisions affecting their teams or circles. Around 70 per cent of its workforce are self-employed, receiving £17 to £21 per hour out of a billing rate of around £24 in early 2024. Although high compared to agency wages, this equates to an employee rate of just £12 to £15, since self-employed people must cover their own pension, holiday and sick pay, plus other overheads and risks.

Equal Care faces similar obstacles to other non-profits: low hourly prices offered by local authorities; difficulty and delay for clients in arranging personal budgets; and difficulty building up to a sufficient scale to support organisational overheads and client choices. All these have impeded its ambition of expansion into North-east London. Their experiences highlight the challenge of enabling community-based co-production at the scale required for financial sustainability. In Calderdale, rapid growth to a turnover level of around £1 million per year with at least 80 care workers is needed to break even. More community volunteers and a faster build-up of client numbers for a non-profit enterprise could perhaps be achieved by partnership with an anchor organisation such as a large community centre or seniors' organisation.

How can non-profit providers achieve a larger scale? One route is finding ways to increase take-up of personal budgets and streamline the process for arranging them. Another is changes in commissioning practices, to facilitate easier entry into the council contract market. Greater Manchester has developed a strategy to promote cooperatives in many sectors, supporting them through changes in public sector commissioning and procurement practices. One ambition is to bring freelancers together into groups for effective tendering.

One non-profit that has expanded in the council contract market is Be Caring, based in Newcastle since 2004 (Westhall and Hughes, 2019). This employee-owned social enterprise with 800 home-carers is the largest provider of homecare to councils in the

Newcastle area. It works mostly with seniors, and also provides supported accommodation to some younger people. Hourly pay is above the NLW, but the main advantage for workers is a range of flexible contract types, with payment either by shift or by visit, and training for career progression through a partnership with Sunderland College.

Another example of a large-scale social enterprise in the care sector is PossAbilities,[19] an employee-controlled Community Interest Company founded by former Rochdale Council workers in 2014. By 2019 they had 600 staff and a £15 million turnover, providing day opportunities, respite care and short breaks, and supported accommodation to young people with learning disabilities and older people with dementia. In leaving the council, the workers hoped to achieve better care with greater control by users, and higher pay. However, improved wages are constrained by the low prices offered in council contracts, despite the Community Interest Company's considerable scale. This example suggests that the route to better pay may be through use of personal budgets rather than large contracts.

North West Care Coop,[20] based in Chester, helps people obtain and use personal budgets. It brings disabled people together in user-cooperatives and employs personal assistants for them. They have a choice of personnel and services, without the headache of managing the paperwork which many seniors find difficult, as do those with learning disabilities. The user-cooperative concept is also useful to commission collective provision; if one person wants an art class or a regular minibus trip to go shopping, it may not exist; but a group can finance it together.

Outcomes-based commissioning and the Buurtzorg model

Considerable economies have also been achieved by changing the way homecare is commissioned and organised. One cost-saving measure is 'outcomes-based commissioning' in which the care plan is defined in terms of desired results rather than a specific task list. Several UK areas have adopted this, including Leeds, Hertfordshire

---

[19] Possabilities, www.possabilities.org.uk
[20] North West Care Coop, https://nwcarecoop.co.uk/

and Wales, which offer useful 'good practice' documentation.[21] The homecare worker decides with the client what tasks need doing to achieve the planned goals. This can save a significant proportion of homecare costs (Cavendish, 2022).

Improved quality of care outcomes at reduced cost has been achieved by the 'Buurtzorg model', developed from around 2007 by a Dutch not-for-profit provider of that name. It features small flexible teams of highly qualified care workers, serving 40–60 patients. They bring together a 'care team' of relatives, friends or neighbours who work with the care worker to achieve the patient's desired outcomes. Seeing the same workers consistently helps the client and informal helpers develop understanding and trust. The aim is to achieve patient self-management as far as possible, improving care worker autonomy and reducing bureaucracy (Cavendish, 2022).

In Scotland, six areas ran a trial of the Buurtzorg model, based in doctors' surgeries (Healthcare Improvement Scotland, 2019). Staffed by nurses working with social care staff, they focused on health issues. The main gains were found to be in reducing hospital admissions, and in the quality of care as experienced by clients. A further pilot in Cambridgeshire is described in Chapter 7.

The Buurtzorg model and outcomes-based commissioning are ways to integrate formal services with help from friends and community projects, drawing on these resources for preventive and ancillary forms of support which can motivate people to sustain normal activities, or return to them after a medical crisis, reducing the risk of further decline.

Cutting costs but not wages: care homes and the alternatives

In early 2024, average costs per week per residential care place for seniors are £800, and £1,078 for nursing care.[22] Most European

---

[21] See Leeds City Council (2018); Hertfordshire Care Providers Association's 'Connected Lives' resource page, https://www.hcpa.info/connectedlives/; Welsh National Commissioning Board (2017)

[22] Cost in December 2023, from Age UK website, www.ageuk.org.uk

countries including the UK have been trying to move away from costly institutional care for some years.

The residential care sector has become very unstable, with several large chains of homes closing in recent years because of financial difficulties (Walker, 2021). Low local authority fees have been blamed for this. But a large proportion of private care home fees enter shareholders' pockets (Scottish Trades Union Congress, 2022). Financialisation of the sector has led to investment returns of 10 to 12 per cent, with complex layers of ownership and much tax evasion (Lyall, 2017; Pollock, 2021). Often the real estate has been bought by a separate company and rented or sold on mortgage to the operating arm. Large profits are then extracted by the real estate company while the actual provider of care is financially squeezed. Except for small-scale homes mainly for people with learning difficulties,[23] non-profit residential care is a minor and declining part of the sector – around 13 per cent of beds in England (Campbell, 2019) and 11 per cent in Scotland (Scottish Government, 2021b).

To buy up residential homes or build new ones would be hugely expensive. An alternative may be integrating provision within extra-care housing, where larger schemes could have some nursing care accommodation. In the United States, where extra-care housing establishments are described as 'assisted living', many have specialised facilities for memory care.[24] Extra-care housing, home adaptations or 'shared lives' may be suitable alternatives to residential care for many people. Sheltered and specialist housing for seniors and for disabled people can save councils and the NHS thousands of pounds per year per resident (ADASS, 2024).

Conclusion

The cost estimates presented here illustrate the difficulties of financing adequate care quickly on a large scale, particularly going

---

[23] For example, in the Suffolk Micro-enterprise directory, see https://www.communitycatalysts.co.uk/smallgoodstuff/subsite/suffolk/
[24] Forbes Health website, 2023, https://health.usnews.com/best-senior-living/assisted-living/articles/dementia-care-in-assisted-living-homes; and the Alzheimer's Association, 2023, https://alzheimersdisease.net/living/what-senior-housing-is-right

into the 2030s as care demand rises, due to population ageing and increased numbers of younger disabled people. But reducing charges would cost much less than the biggest challenge of just providing enough formal care at adequate wages and high standards. Expressed as an *addition* to the net local authority adult care budget in 2022/3, which was £22.3 billion from local councils,[25] rough estimates derived from Health Foundation (2023) are:

- £3.4 billion as the current cost of removing local authority charges, without improving quality or workers' pay, or extending services to cover unmet needs. This would help self-funders of council-arranged care, rather than those with greatest need for care.
- £5.3 million to make care free as part of an expanded service covering some unmet needs, but without improving carers' wages.
- Up to £7 billion to abolish charges while paying care workers £15 per hour.

Adequate expansion of the service and help for *unpaid* carers would cost:

- Around £30 billion for meeting the needs of *everyone* eligible and likely to apply for residential or homecare according to Care Act standards for 'severe' needs, if care workers were paid a minimum of £15 per hour (based on the calculations in Appendix A). This is before deducting any user charges.
- About £16.2 billion gross, or £5.2 billion net, to transform Carer's Allowance and Attendance Allowance into an employment income for unpaid carers, paying full-time carers for, say, 20 hours per week.
- Further costs of assessment, day services, respite care and home adaptations also need to be added.

The first two figures total over £35.2 billion *in addition to* the current adult care budget. That cannot be found overnight,

---

[25] https://www.gov.uk/government/statistics/local-authority-revenue-expenditure-and-financing-2023-24-budget-england/local-authority-revenue-expenditure-and-financing-2023-24-budget-england

nor can enough staff be recruited and trained quickly. But we need to make a start immediately, particularly since formal care demand is expected to increase by over half during the next 15 years.[26]

The biggest elements in a desirable care reform budget would come from meeting unmet need and raising care workers' wages to the level needed to maintain the workforce. Reducing charges requires much less than the task of providing *enough* formal care. Scottish experience suggests that making personal care free raises homecare demand only slightly, while reducing demand for residential care.

The cost of expanding formal care would be partly offset by substantial savings to the NHS and some extra income tax yield. Better access to care would mean fewer emergency hospital admissions and easier hospital discharge. Some informal carers would do more paid work. Advocates of larger care spending have argued that a substantial portion of care staff wages returns to the government in taxes paid and benefits saved. However, this is true only if the total earned by newly recruited care workers is more than they earned in the UK before – that is, if they are new immigrants, or economically inactive, or previously had lower incomes. It has been argued that there are also job creation benefits – but creating jobs means finding people to fill vacancies, currently a major problem of the sector.

There are many untapped sources of tax revenue, of which Appendix A provides examples. But there are also many pressing demands for public services and cash benefits that will compete with the care budget over several years. As inequality soars (Wernham and Brewer, 2022), the case for redistributive taxation and better benefits grows ever stronger. Although there will be difficult choices between competing demands, the fiscal capacity of the economy is considerable for any administration with the courage to redistribute wealth.

---

[26] Hu et al (2020) estimated a 72 per cent rise in the population aged at least 85 between 2018 and 2038. Applying this same annual rate to the period 2024/5 to 2039/40 gives 54 per cent. Continuing the trend line estimated by the Health Foundation up to 2031/2 (Health Foundation, 2018) to 2039/40 gives 58 per cent.

Costs could be somewhat reduced by supply-side changes. Use of residential care, by seniors at least, could be replaced by more homecare, which most of them would prefer. Some small savings in unit costs, and considerable improvement in quality, can be found from non-profit providers. Cooperatives and micro-enterprises, working with personal budget users, could provide higher wages for care workers more easily than corporate providers. They can work with a slightly lower margin between billing rate and wage than corporate agencies, especially if operating very locally which cuts down travel time. They offer opportunities for improving the quality of care by better personalisation and user control, and for teamwork with informal carers and volunteers.

Personal budgets for homecare offer more flexibility in choice and management of care than a fixed 'care package'. They allow people to spend their ration of care time as they wish, avoiding a rigid definition of what tasks are covered. But their complex administration presents barriers for some people, including many seniors. An intermediary organisation like North West Care Coop may be needed to increase the take-up of personal budgets. Councils need to allow personal assistants the same hourly rate as agency workers; currently they are often lower.

The way in which local authorities approach care and support offers considerable opportunity for reducing need, particularly for residential care, but also for *any* formal support. Preventive action is crucial to forestall declining health in middle and older age. Chapter 7 attempts to show its potential not only for improving quality of life, but to contain growth of the care budget and make reducing charges more feasible.

Resources for free care are inevitably limited; choices need to be made about how to distribute it according to financial need, clinical need and load for unpaid carers. Options for a partial, gradual lifting of care charges might be:

- Making co-payments for care depend on the level of need; above the minimum asset level and minimum income guarantee level at which co-payments would begin, people would contribute to the first so many hours of care per week. If they needed more, the extra hours would be free. This is similar to the Welsh weekly £120 cap. But a clear inflation-proofing

method needs to be defined for users, workers and their employers. Perhaps ring-fenced care funding could be indexed to the Real Living Wage. Hopefully, over time, it would rise faster, and the cap would fall, allowing more hours to be free and less hours to be co-paid. The initial size of the weekly cap is obviously debatable. It would help more people sooner than the now abandoned plan for a lifetime cap of £86,000.
- Increasing personal budgets free of charge, for people who rely heavily on an unpaid carer. The main carer would be allowed to accept the money as a wage or pay someone else.
- Means testing, if retained at all, should be as simple as possible. Higher taxes on everyone with higher income or wealth seem fairer than a 'tax on disability' – self-funding for those wealthy people who have the misfortune to need any.

Further research is needed to see how these proposals could be combined, estimating their costs and behavioural effects.

Whatever system of user charges and their reduction is adopted, there are also choices about how much subsidy should be reserved for other important objectives: staff training, investment in new provider capacity, day services, assessment and advice, preventive health measures, and carer support.

Support structures for isolated seniors and for family carers need to be greatly improved to maintain active, healthy lifestyles, sustain and widen their social networks, and provide them with more help from friends and neighbours. These topics are addressed in Chapters 5 and 6.

5

Widening the caring circle: towards a caring economy

Introduction

Chapter 4 has shown how challenging it would be to meet all of the care shortage by expanding formal care. The vast bulk of care hours comes from the unpaid sector, so it needs to expand at least as fast as the population in need. Hopefully it can help to dampen the rising trend of need for formal care, by supporting people at an early stage of their difficulties and helping them to stay in good health – and obviously happier – for longer. There is a need to widen the circle of support, especially for isolated seniors and family carers. This chapter shows how friends and neighbours can help with that part of 'moderate needs' which involves instrumental activities of daily living rather than activities of daily living, things like going out, shopping, housework and advice on digital communications. These are often unsupported in the current care shortage.

Previous chapters presented a quantitative perspective; how many people are needed for tasks measured in hours. We need this to define the scale of the care deficit, but it is important not to obscure the qualitative perspective of care as a social activity and a relationship. This chapter first examines the qualitative and ethical basis for a vision of 'widening the caring circle', outlining the central values of solidarity – 'relational care', 'politics of compassion', the 'commons of care', mutual support and co-production – which form foundational concepts for engaging the community to address the care deficit. It then attempts to identify the first building block of a 'caring economy' – supportive personal networks – and how community projects have worked to widen them. Chapter 6 will then examine some other important building blocks for widening the caring circle: mutual aid groups, timebanks, community unions and traditional volunteer groups.

Beyond the family, the first source of support in older age is friends. They are sources of practical help, emotional support, and sometimes information and advice. Help of the kind that homecare provides is only one part of the support seniors want. The desire for company, social connection and activities outside the home features prominently in surveys about unmet need (Age UK, 2018). It is also an important need of intensive carers, as evidenced by the comments from the Campsbourne Collective described in this chapter. Some people find sociability and helpful friends for themselves; others do not, and may need a boost from organisations of some kind to help them connect with others – a lunch club, a sports or music group, a religious congregation or regular community centre meet-ups. This chapter discusses the successes and failures of two major projects which have attempted to build supportive social networks through bringing people together for social activities with some element of mutual aid – the Cares Family and Circles.

Social activity is important not only to improve people's quality of life, but because, through maintaining health, it reduces the long-term demand for care. With much research showing that lonely people are more likely to suffer health problems in older age, preventing isolation has become a major aspect of preventive health measures in the UK. Mental stimulation through participating in more social and cultural activity is thought to reduce the risk of dementia (Jisca et al, 2015; Cunyoen et al, 2016). Loneliness has been linked to coronary heart disease (Hemingway and Marmot, 1999) and functional decline (Avlund et al, 2004). With these problems in mind, 'social prescribers' attached to doctors' practices have been established to help people find clubs and classes where they can meet new people and acquire new friends. 'Social prescribing' can also encourage exercise to preserve physical capacity, through walking groups and yoga, pilates or dance sessions that are also sociable.

Care as a relationship rather than a set of tasks

As well as help with 'activities of daily living', people also need emotional support, listening and friendship. Occasionally isolated individuals may find this from their formal home-carers. But in current conditions of staff shortage and strained budgets, this is inevitably rare. Formal homecare, at least in its current British form, is narrowly task-oriented, based on the Care Act assessment of what is needed to support hygiene and survival. Care workers must largely limit their attention to tasks listed in the care plan – washing, dressing, serving food – then rush to the next client, leaving little time to talk. They are often conflicted about having so little time to establish the more human relationship with clients that they want.[1]

Care as a *relationship* is central to the work of Kartupelis (2021) on 'relational care'. She calls for radical change in the care industry – for recognition of human interdependence; the need to do things *with* people rather than *to or for* them, focusing on them being respected in a framework of love and trust. This requires sustained, supportive relationships, offering people meaning and purpose in their lives, and perhaps above all, more time. Although Kartupelis' work focuses on formal care, her approach resonates with other recent writing about the need for a 'caring community' in which care becomes a generalised collective responsibility.

Segal and her co-authors in the Care Collective (Chatzidikis et al, 2020) defined care very broadly as care for each other, whatever our status, nationality, health or circumstances, and care for the planet. They envisioned 'a model of universal care; the ideal of a society in which care is placed front and centre on every scale of life' (Chatzidikis et al, 2020: 19). An important aspect of this is mutual aid as a vehicle for informal care:

---

[1] See Caroline Weimar's speech to a seminar at Birkbeck University, London, in 2020, https://www.youtube.com/watch?v=F0PWKlZmDmM&list=PL2Fy-5oxIlb72tRO-O1XN1-Ahklep88D2&index=18; and the video, 'Homecare Worker Stories', made as part of the 'Paid Homecare work in London: invisible work, invisible knowledges' project in 2020, https://www.youtube.com/watch?v=_iTuSah5RXo

> Communities based on caregiving and caretaking provide each other with mutual forms of support ... local mutual aid groups in Europe and elsewhere during the COVID-19 pandemic have been an excellent example of how such neighbourly support networks can expand. ... Caring for a wide range of people by offering forms of support beyond immediate kinship networks is one hallmark of a caring community. (Chatzidikis et al, 2020: 47)

Mutual support in this context refers to instrumental help, friendship and information; from the phone call perhaps to the kitchen table, but not bedroom and bathroom tasks. Personal care, by contrast, is clearly defined as the territory of formal care: 'all care work should be properly resourced and democratically organised, not left to the free labour of strangers' (Chatzidikis et al, 2020: 43). Restricted by lockdown rules and the need for social distancing, mutual-aiders during the COVID-19 pandemic could not enter homes. But in the longer term, neighbourly support networks could have wider roles without crossing the boundary into personal care. Chapter 6 considers how timebanks and mutual aid groups could do this.

The Care Collective critiques the current form of formal care in the UK, since 'marketising care foregrounds self-interest and instrumentality in every sphere of our (uncaring) lives. Inevitably, both the even distribution of care work and its quality decline' (Chatzidikis et al, 2020: 77). They call for replacing a market logic, focused on impersonal delivery of fixed services for money, with a care logic which involves mutuality and patience, embedding the exchange relationship in a framework of compassion and respect. Whereas Kartupelis sets out a 'business case' for commercial providers to adopt a 'relational' approach, the Care Collective argues for largely non-profit forms of formal care provision, through the state, cooperatives or social enterprises.

The politics of compassion and the commons of care

A closely related concept to the 'caring community' is the 'politics of compassion'. It is distinct from charity, because it embraces the necessity of a struggle for social change: Lynne Segal states that a compassionate politics of care 'is quite distinct from benevolence or pity'. She argues for 'persuading people to broaden their compassion to value all the ties that bind us, near and far, and to fight for the social and economic policies which might provide good lives for all on a habitable planet' (Segal, 2023: 227–8). Segal cites the view of Pragna Patel, an activist in the well-known Asian women's group in West London Southall Black Sisters, that 'compassion must also connect with a vision of, and struggle for, comprehensive social justice'. This means empowering disabled and older people by helping them to gain voice, political and social agency and inclusion.

Both Segal and the Care Collective base their work loosely on the feminist ethics of care. Tronto (2005, 2013) characterises care ethics as having five core values: compassion, responsibility, competence, responsiveness to the needs of the other and solidarity. The last of these involves trust, respect, communication and working together to address the need for care on a collective basis. The ethics of care requires listening, acting responsively and responsibly to the context of relationships, attempting to understand the cared-for person's needs and emotions (Noddings, 2013). Seen in a collective context, these values resonate with the growing emphasis on the co-production of care (Beresford and Carr, 2012), in which service users and professionals work together to develop the 'menu' of support options, based on the principle that 'those affected are the best placed to help design it'.[2]

Under the title 'Care as Commons', Thomas Allan[3] critiques marketised formal care in terms similar to Kartupelis and Segal: 'Care is a relationship built upon love, shared vulnerability, emotional proximity, and responsibility. It is not a scarce commodity that must be packaged, before being "delivered" as

---

[2] The Involve Foundation, organisational website describing co-production concepts and methods, https://www.involve.org.uk/resource/co-production
[3] Resilience, a blog site, https://www.resilience.org/stories/2020-11-12/care-as-commons-a-brief-introduction/

quickly and as cheaply as possible, like an Amazon order.' He defines the 'commons' as 'shared resources co-governed by its user community' which would be realised 'not only through the logic of contract, but through empathy, trust, reciprocity and mutual support', hoping to 'transcend the pathologies of our current gridlocked "market-state" order'. Allan calls for 'a movement and a framework for care and for society that enables people to live their own definition of dignity; derives from the experience of the caring relation; and emerges through that same shared experience'.

Mutuality involves a recognition of interdependence, rather than a precise concept of reciprocal exchange; according to Kartupelis the 'interdependence' aspect of relational care encompasses a recognition that we need to serve as well as be served. Similarly, Segal refers to Graeber's statement that we all need to be cared for, but we also have a psychological need to care for others, or at least to care for something.[4]

These related elements of the 'caring economy' – the 'commons of care', 'relational care', mutual support and co-production – form the basis of mutual aid groups, which exhibit a combination of altruism, compassion and often, but not always, commitment to social justice and improvement. The term 'mutual' conveys the idea that solidarity requires reciprocity. But in practice, as described in Chapter 6, the mutual aid model corresponds more to the Marxian ambition of 'from each according to his/her ability; to each according to his/her need'.

Some interesting reflections on the needs of informal carers and those they care for, and how community support and formal services might mesh together, came from a community project in Haringey, North London. They illustrate the importance of emotional support and of social relationships in meeting care needs, echoing the concerns of Kartupelis and Segal. The Campsbourne Community Collective emerged from mutual aid

---

[4] David Graeber, 'From Managerial Feudalism to the Revolt of the Caring Classes', talk given to 36th Chaos Communication Congress, 27 December 2019, transcript available at www.opentranscripts.org.

groups on a small council estate and in adjacent higher-income, privately owned housing. This Collective received support from the Open University and some funding from the Institute of Community Studies in 2021 to train a cohort of community-based researchers and develop a resident-led research agenda in close collaboration with the institutions embedded in the estate (a primary school, sheltered and supported living accommodation, migrant advice centre, food bank and the council).[5] Five programmes of research and action were identified, including one on care. Each programme started with a co-creation phase, which brought together local stakeholders including care recipients, paid and unpaid carers, care providers, care activists, researchers and policy makers. This phase identified three priority areas: improvement of early intervention through community systems; better links between hospital discharge systems and home/community environments; and recognition of carers' knowledge and needs.

Following group discussions over several months a small pot of funding from Birkbeck University supported a community engagement project to map paid and unpaid care on the Campsbourne Estate. An arts-based approach involved research with different groups of residents on the estate to produce artworks exploring care practices, needs and priorities, while an interactive art exhibition in the community centre invited the broader community as well as professionals and policy makers to contribute to the conversation.[6] Visitors contributed their thoughts through sticky notes and pictures on display panels, yielding the themes summarised in Boxes 5.1 and 5.2. Many individual comments on the displays emphasised the importance of care as a relationship.

---

[5] Open University, https://oro.open.ac.uk/86336/
[6] A photographic record and other documents are preserved on the Collective's website, https://campsbournecommunitycollective.wordpress.com

Box 5.1: Themes from the Campsbourne Community Collective's exhibition on care

Pressures on carers and cared-for people	What is needed
Time sacrifice/stress	Respite centres and facilities Sharing some regular tasks with community helpers More formal care
Emotional support, friendship, socialising	Social opportunities with other carers Inclusion in community events/friendship networks Formal counselling and advocacy
Managerial responsibility for household; access to services (for example, housing repair, benefits) and household upkeep	Information Better online access; computer skills training Task sharing with community (for example, DIY, shopping) Advocacy
Need for help with physical/medical needs of cared-for person	More formal homecare Easier access to doctor's appointments Training in health and first aid
Money	Higher allowances/benefits Help with energy costs and with grants for insulation or heating systems Information about forms of help

The phrase 'commons of care' also appeared on one of the interactive display panels and resonated widely with residents who attended the exhibition. At the launch event, several residents spoke about their life experiences of caring. Among them, Burçu Kever reflected Segal's concern with the 'politics of compassion', saying that 'care means putting the needs of someone else before your own'. Her speech at the exhibition's launch event (see Appendix C) reflected the complex emotions surrounding this, and carers' need for emotional support.

Box 5.2: Selected comments on the qualities of carers and caring from the Campsbourne project exhibition

What is a carer?

Someone who gives support and takes time out to listen.

Someone who takes time out of their lives to make a difference to someone else.

What do carers do and how do they feel?

Managing and supporting someone with their health care needs and appointments.

Pressure and responsibility to explain care and diagnosis to others.

The constant feeling of guilt and not doing enough.

Feeling alone and unsupported.

Need peer group support and sociability.

Grief at the life you have lost.

What qualities and expertise do carers bring?

Flexibility; advocacy; patience; understanding; the ability to empathise; inclusivity, love, tolerance, patience and a voice; translating across culture and gender; understanding social norms; protection.

The author explored the exhibition's themes in a group interview with four residents: two South Asian, two Black Caribbean and one Kurdish. One, retired, cared for her bedridden husband; two younger women described experiences of parent-care. Another, a full-time mother, faced many years of caring for two disabled children, the oldest just reaching adulthood. All had experienced very poor access to formal care. They had great difficulty knowing what they could ask for or how. Waiting for care assessments took several months. Application procedures for disability benefits were daunting; one (a graduate with perfect English) needed two sessions with an advice worker to complete the 32-page form for her husband's Personal Independence Payment. They lamented the high cost of self-funded care – for example £90 per day for a disabled teenager's day-centre place. Advocacy and help with navigating service systems was a strongly felt need, to help negotiate formal care, medical appointments, a day-centre placement, a housing transfer or home repairs.

Perhaps most importantly, they also emphasised the severe emotional impact of caring responsibilities: isolation, guilt, being unable to switch off thinking about an unending list of tasks, or spend time outside the house. They wanted opportunities to socialise with other carers; a centre where they could drop in to swap experiences and information with each other. Although support from volunteers would be welcome for shopping, perhaps for visiting and short periods of respite care, they stressed the importance of Disclosure and Barring Service (DBS) checks and matching of volunteers to visited people. This would need to take account of language barriers, food culture and interests. Some older people they knew were most reluctant to accept help from strangers; there were issues of privacy and safety.

Some other individual accounts in the exhibition highlighted the extreme stresses of long-term caring. These included difficulties of *negotiating* formal care from services which are short of money, staff, assessment capacity, and flexibility in relation to autism and complex needs. They called for good information, respite, a listening ear and mutual peer support with other carers. They also emphasised carer poverty, due to being unable to work for many years. All this resonates with lived experiences of parents who become life-long carers for adult children, as illustrated in a video from the campaigning group End Social Care Disgrace, of which Jo's story (Appendix C) is a partial transcript.[7]

Based in a community centre, the Campsbourne Community Collective saw carer support very much in a group setting. Help to individuals would be welcome, with the important provisos about vetting, matching and DBS checks. But their main emphasis was on the importance of socialising, gathering information to share and pressing for better formal services.

---

[7] End Social Care Disgrace, video recording of a meeting on Fair Deal for Carers, https://www.youtube.com/watch?v=8lN_Xxf84MY

What can friends and neighbours contribute to informal care?

Turning to how the circle of support might be widened for individual seniors, with what kinds of tasks do people need more support? What do non-relatives actually do and what tasks are suitable for them to take on? Appendix B shows survey evidence from the English Longitudinal Study of Ageing and the Health Survey of England about how tasks are typically divided between formal care services and different kinds of informal helpers: partners, daughters, sons, other relatives, friends and neighbours. Non-kin play a minor role; though hopefully this could be improved by more social interaction, perhaps in the context of mutual aid groups and similar projects, but also through just widening and deepening personal friendships.

There is a spectrum of different type of care tasks, ranging from those for which professional help is most commonly used, through tasks generally done by close relatives to ones which are shared by non-relatives and more distant kin. Statistical evidence suggests a gradient of intimacy and specialised competence which affects the 'division of labour'. Most seniors would prefer bedroom and bathroom assistance – defined as 'personal care' – to be offered by their partner if they have one, or by an adult daughter (for women) or son (for men). If a suitable relative is unavailable, lacks strength, or is over-burdened, they will turn to formal services.

The information on who does what in Appendix B reflects the 'gradient' of intimacy between personal care and other activities. Bedroom and bathroom activities, helping someone serve and cut up food, and help with medication, require an intimate or a homecare worker. Unpaid help with these – the first five tasks listed in Figure B2 (Appendix B) – mainly falls to partners, daughters and sons. The need for formal services to support bedroom and bathroom tasks is irreducible except in two ways. One is health improvements; the second is housing design and adaptations.

Seniors' children – particularly daughters who are most frequently involved – often feel a conflict between maintaining their paid job and caring for their parent(s). They may experience a need for formal help even when the parent(s) do not. Naturally, having a paid worker entails loss of privacy and family autonomy;

the receiver of care may resent that, even when accepting an outside helper becomes important for their relatives. But relatives may sometimes face tasks beyond their strength or experience. Many women are smaller than their father or male partner; helping him into bed or pushing a wheelchair can be difficult to manage alone. There is also a risk that the caring relative(s) may suffer harm from lack of sleep or general stress, which is not necessarily measured by how many hours someone spends caring.

The lot of overloaded family members could be alleviated somewhat if some tasks were more widely shared. The contribution of non-relatives to informal care is largely for instrumental activities of daily living-related tasks like shopping, gardening, housework, home maintenance and offering lifts. Another important need is supporting seniors' capacity for 'managing paperwork and paying bills'. All too often, this now must be done not on paper but online. Help with computer and mobile phone operations has become a major social need for seniors, many of whom have great difficulty with internet use (Age UK, 2024).

An illustration of the scale of these needs for non-family help is that in a typical street of 200 homes, there will be around 540 people, of whom around 100 will be over 65. Nine or ten of these seniors will feel unable to go out much on their own. They may need a lift to the high street or the cinema, or a helping arm to cross a busy road into the park. They might welcome help with spring-cleaning and moving furniture, minor repairs to taps or windows; with heavy garden work like digging, grass cutting or tree pruning; or stepladder jobs like changing light bulbs or taking down curtains for cleaning. As many as 13 might be frustrated that things they need to pay for or find out about are online, when they have great difficulty with their mobile phones. Perhaps they can only use wi-fi and the bigger screen of a computer in the public library – which is too far for some of them to walk.

Some of the heaviest loads fall to those who are carers for a partner or an adult child. The seniors needing support will include some of these. Additionally, there will be around 25 younger households in the 200 homes with a disabled person and often their family carer, all needing to feel integrated into the community, able to go out, live life to the fullest extent possible, and preserve their dignity and independence.

Personal networks: loneliness and help from friends

What sort of friendship patterns are most likely to lead to support in older age? And what kinds of people are most at risk of social isolation? Company and emotional support come most easily from intimates, who may be either family or friends; people with whom one shares common interests, frequent contact and awareness of each other's history. But some people's relatives are few or live far away; families may also be conflicted and stressed. Relationships of choice, whether with kin or non-kin, are a key protection against loneliness (Holt-Lunstad et al, 2010; Gray and Worlledge, 2018).

Network theory provides a body of important research about how different kinds of personal contacts provide people with practical and emotional support. Studies of social network types have found that people with the most personal support, and feelings of security about help in time of difficulty, are those with substantial mixed or 'diverse' personal networks, including relatives, neighbours and personal friends (Wenger et al, 1996; Fiori et al, 2018). Relatives tend to be the most committed to providing support over long periods. But as mentioned in Chapter 3, single seniors without adult children nearby lack access to family support – unless from a niece, nephew, grandchild or sibling, which is much less common. Sometimes close friends may help more than distant relatives in times of sickness or difficulty; the gay community has set pathbreaking examples of care-sharing beyond the family, as noted by the Care Collective (Chatzidikis et al, 2020). Friends or neighbours may also have access to skills or information which your own family does not – such as DIY expertise or detailed knowledge of local services or the benefits system. They may provide links to other contacts; possibly across boundaries of occupational or local knowledge, ethnicity or language. Often termed a 'bridging' or 'linking' form of social capital (Litwin and Shiovitz-Ezra, 2015), contacts of this kind may be particularly helpful to migrants from other countries or regions. Hence the 'mixed' type of social network, with non-family contacts from several sources, tends to offer more kinds of support than a family-based one. In Appendix C, Elfrida, Margaret and Hyacinth are examples of people with mixed or diverse networks.

Personal network quality connects with care and support needs in at least three different ways. Firstly, if people *feel* lonely, this indicates that their personal network is too small, or provides insufficient empathy and emotional support. They need more contacts, possibly of different kinds, or to relate to them in different ways. Perhaps they are shy or withdrawn after a crisis, sickness or bereavement. Perhaps their closest friends have died or moved and are hard to replace. Secondly, some people don't feel lonely because they do have close confidantes, but these confidantes don't provide practical support – because of their own age or infirmity, or they lack the right skills, time or knowledge. Relying on a very small network, however close and helpful, also risks that they may move or become sick – or even die, which is why seniors need to know younger people. Thirdly, loneliness may lead to depression, lack of self-care and exercise, and also insufficient mental stimulation which is associated in seniors with a greater risk of memory loss (James et al, 2011). A link between loneliness and poor health features in numerous research studies in the UK and elsewhere (Holt-Lunstad et al, 2010; Iecovitch et al, 2011). The direction of causation is not always clear; poor health and loneliness may worsen each other in a vicious circle. Because of its impact on health status and the long-term need for care, keeping people active and engaged with others has become an important preventive objective in current health and care practice.

Wenger (1994) found, in a longitudinal study of rural Wales, that the personal network type which most protected against feelings of loneliness was a 'wider, community focussed one', with many contacts including relatives both near and living far away, friends, neighbours and some organisational involvements. This type of network appears to be associated with higher income levels. Scharf and de Jong Gierveld (2008) found that it is relatively rare in low-income urban neighbourhoods in Britain, where loneliness is higher than the UK average. They also found that perceived neighbourhood quality affects how lonely people feel.

Cattell (2001) developed a typology of personal networks which includes one described as 'solidaristic' and similar to Wenger's 'wide community focussed network'. Her study, of two East London social housing estates, suggests that it is not confined to higher income groups. People with 'solidaristic' networks have many different groups of people to ask for support – family, friends, neighbours and organisations. This helps them withstand stress and also access information easily. Through many and varied contacts, they are aware of other people's problems, and get a sense of satisfaction from helping others.

Cattell also describes a 'heterogeneous' network type in which individuals meet their contacts through voluntary organisations; people who may be unlike them in occupation, gender, age or ethnicity. They have fewer close bonds but relatively good access to information from this large variety of contacts, for example about benefits and health services. They can pass this on to friends and relatives. Thus, networks derived from voluntary groups can be an important community resource.

Other network types found in Cattell's study included the 'homogeneous' one consisting of a locally resident extended family plus a small number of friends and neighbours. They had friends mainly drawn from school, work and sport clubs. Many older, long-standing resident seniors had this kind of network. It may leave them isolated if their local relatives disperse. People with 'traditional' networks, based mainly just on the extended family, had even fewer contacts. Finally, the 'excluded' network type, with few local contacts of any kind, contained newcomers (including some refugees), lone parents and some isolated seniors.

Cattell makes an important point about the isolation of carers; their need for sociability and for 'bridging social capital' that gives access to important sources of peer-group knowledge about services and the experience of others. This was echoed in the exhibition and discussions of the Campsbourne Collective, mentioned earlier.

The author used British Household Panel Survey data to study the effect of membership of various types of voluntary organisations and interaction with neighbours (Gray, 2009). Sports clubs and religious organisations seemed to improve social support, although several other types of voluntary organisation did not. The influence of sports clubs may reflect a 'virtuous circle' of relative fitness, social and physical activity, and remaining fit and connected to a social circle. With religious organisations, what counted was regular meeting with the congregation. Religious congregations often set up telephone contact circles for seniors to sustain their wellbeing. However, voluntary and religious groups had less influence than relationships with neighbours. These were measured through an index of 'neighbourhood attachment' developed by Li et al (2005), which combined the answers to British Household Panel Survey questions on five aspects of neighbour contact; whether people feel similar to their neighbours and talk to them regularly; whether friends in the neighbourhood mean a lot; whether advice is locally available; and whether neighbours swap favours with each other.

Informal relationships may be more important to mutual support than membership of organisations. However, voluntary work or participation in organisations may help people develop the confidence and 'people skills' to make friends with strangers. This was evident from survey work about life in seniors' retirement housing estates (Gray and Worlledge, 2018). People there who had been involved in voluntary work, clubs or organisations in earlier life, or had held civic office, had more sense of feeling supported in times of difficulty, including by their *current* neighbours. This study also showed the value of bringing seniors together with neighbours; where the estate had relatively more organised social activities, more people reported making friends among their neighbours, and expected that someone would help with food shopping or laundry if they were ill. These findings confirm a study of American seniors, which suggested that group attendance *generates* friendships, rather than simply being its outcome (Litwin and Shiovitz-Ezra, 2015).

However, opportunities to meet others, although a *necessary* condition of developing helpful and satisfying social networks, are not a *sufficient* condition. Continuity and frequency of contact are preconditions of friendship turning into support; normative expectations and reciprocity also play a part (Keating et al, 2003). Formal group activity is just a springboard which may or may not lead to supportive friendships. But these may not provide attachment figures or close confidantes. In particular, Van Baarsen (2002) found that neither emotional nor practical support from personal networks alleviated emotional loneliness following partner loss. However, people did feel less lonely if they had relatively high self-esteem, which may develop from positive social contacts. Befriending schemes offering visits or phone calls from volunteers may help isolated individuals to generate the confidence and motivation to reach out to new social circles. But just talking may not be enough; accompanying the befriended person on an outing or group activity is needed to develop or restore their confidence to go out and socialise (Cattan et al, 2005).

A complex interaction exists between neighbourhood, personal networks and a sense of loneliness or feeling unsupported. People will get to know more of their neighbours if they can see them easily and feel they have something in common. However, neighbours may or may not be trusted to help when needed – to do shopping if you are sick, or support you during a health or domestic emergency. Neighbours may not always share your own interests and values enough to become *friends*. American research has found feelings of exclusion and powerlessness by people who feel their neighbours are wealthier than they are (Ross et al, 2001). This may occur where low-income renters and wealthier home-owners live close together.

Housing and neighbourhood design influences how much people see their neighbours. It may be hard to know who lives on a busy street with many non-residents walking about. In a courtyard or gated community, almost anyone you see probably lives there, so neighbours are more easily recognised. Low back garden fences invite eye contact and chats; so do encounters in lifts, shared entrances and stairways. But even if people see their neighbours, they may not trust them if the area has a reputation for crime or there are problems about noise, vandalism or litter. Fear of crime deters people from going out, especially in the evenings when they have most chance of meeting others from different age groups in community centres, cafes or pubs. Community stability helps people to get to know neighbours and improves levels of trust. Owner-occupiers move on average once in around 20 years, though with much variation between region and property type. Areas with a high proportion of private renters, who move much more frequently, have relatively low stability. Areas with good community facilities – shops, cafes, community centres, well-kept parks and popular schools, obviously attract people to stay, so that neighbour relationships and community organisations grow.

The value of intergenerational contacts is an important aspect of making supportive friends. Seniors need friends who will still be alive and hopefully fit when they themselves reach their late 80s, the age when many people become less active and more dependent. A study of the London borough of Camden in 2005 (Gray, 2006), interviewed helpers at over-50s clubs which the council had set up in community centres and sheltered housing schemes. These attracted several volunteers in their 50s and early 60s who ran social activities for the older ones. The importance of this form of support from younger seniors to older seniors was confirmed in the retirement housing study mentioned earlier (Gray, 2015; Gray and Worlledge, 2018). All too often, residents' groups which ran social gatherings became dormant when their leaders died or became too age-affected to continue. Leaders were difficult to replace, because due to the housing shortage, intake of new residents was increasingly restricted to the most dependent, so few active people in their 60s could come in.

Housing providers can help to generate informal contacts between neighbours, developing peer support and mutual aid. Examples in relation to retirement housing are provided in Blood and Pannell (2012), Callaghan et al (2008), Darton et al (2008), and in the 'good neighbour' schemes reported in Hanover Housing Group (2009). Through music events, IT help and shared gardening projects, Hanover Housing has also sought to promote intergenerational contacts between residents and volunteers from outside their retirement housing schemes. Such initiatives need not be confined to *retirement* housing. Rochdale Borough Housing in the Greater Manchester area is a major partner in the Rochdale Circle, which has become a national model for generating social contacts between seniors.

Projects to build supportive friendships: 'Circles' and the Cares Family

The last 15 years has seen the foundation, development and partial collapse of two important movements to help seniors build friendships and mutual support; the Circles projects and the Cares 'Family', each with a presence in several cities.

The Circles movement began in the South London borough of Southwark in 2009. As related by its founder Hilary Cottam (2019), it started with phone circles, bringing together seniors who wanted friendship. It developed rapidly into a staffed office with council funding. In Cottam's words, it was 'part social club, part concierge service, and part cooperative self-help group', responding to three needs for a good older age:

> [S]omeone to take care of the little things – to go up a ladder and fix the light bulb before you fall over in the dark; good company – people who share your interests and with whom you feel at ease; and a sense of purpose and the support necessary to make the shifts into a different ways of living as our interests and life phases change. (Cottam, 2019: 154)

Using a digital database of members' leisure interests and skills for helping each other, the four staff serviced a membership of 1,000 people who each paid £30 per year. Staff and members together organised social events and linked people with volunteers for practical help with DIY, gardening, shopping, lifts and support after hospital discharge. Friendships developed, which provided some of these tasks without going through the request system. Volunteers also came from outside the membership; neighbours of members or people attached to other volunteer organisations. Thus Southwark Circle addressed both loneliness and instrumental support, reducing the need for formal care and supporting members' health and wellbeing.

The model attracted enthusiasm from some other local authorities. Cottam's team sought start-up funding of £750,000 over three years for each area. Savings in formal care services, National Health Service and other public service costs of over £2 million were expected during this period. But despite its substantial scale and membership fees, Southwark Circle was unable to break even when council support ended. It closed in 2014. Suffolk Circle, founded in 2011 with £680,000 of county council funding, also failed to achieve financial viability, possibly because it duplicated some existing work by Age UK and Suffolk Family Carers. Before it closed in 2014, it had 2,000 members and had offered 1,500 hours of practical help.[8] The Nottingham Circle, founded in 2011, has also now closed its company. A social

---

[8] BBC News item, 'Suffolk Circle closing', 14 March 2014, https://www.bbc.co.uk/news/uk-england-suffolk-26585520

audit report attached to its Companies House return of 2012 recorded 342 members and a considerable volume of practical help offered at between £10 and £15 per hour, for which the helpers were paid. Southwark Circle and Suffolk Circle also operated a person-to-person request system for help with specific tasks, but unlike Nottingham, volunteers were not paid.

The biggest success of the Circle model has been in Rochdale, Greater Manchester, which survives in 2024. The Heywood, Middleton and Rochdale Circle was founded in 2012 with start-up funding of £150,000 over three years from Rochdale Borough Housing and the borough council. With other grants from charitable organisations, and sales of services, total income was around £320,000 in 2022/3. In February 2024 there were around 1,000 members, each paying £30 annually. Through its social events for people over 50, the Circle helps to avoid loneliness and develop friendships that may lead to practical support. Volunteers operate the highly successful taxi service; by paying drivers just for expenses, it charges customers well below market taxi fares. Many drivers are from younger age groups, which generates some intergenerational contacts for members. The taxi service helps to cross-subsidise the overall overheads of the Rochdale Circle.

An evaluation survey of 200 members (Rochdale Circle, nd) found that two-thirds had joined just for social reasons. A majority said their health and wellbeing had improved, and 14 per cent visited their doctor less often. Almost 72 per cent had made new friends, on average seven each. A third of members joined at least partly to obtain practical support; the cheap taxi service was particularly popular. But apart from this volunteer driver scheme, person-to-person help within the Rochdale Circle depends on the friendships members make.

The Rochdale model inspired the foundation of the Haringey Circle in North London, in 2019. It had initial funding from the local council for two part-time staff, later supplemented by charitable grants of £30,000. Haringey's grant funding so far has been under £150 per member, compared to over £300 in Rochdale. Its expansion was hampered by the COVID-19 pandemic, and by a high annual subscription rate of £48. For social events it competed with another older people's group which cost merely £10 per year, and the University of the Third Age at £38 in 2023 (since reduced). In late 2023, when 370 people either were or had been members, Haringey Circle abolished subscriptions and now seeks to cover costs from charitable funding. It has changed from a Community Interest Company to a charity, which makes fundraising easier.

During the COVID-19 pandemic, the borough council asked Haringey Circle to recruit volunteers for medicine delivery to self-isolating people. Over 40 volunteers made 900 deliveries, sometimes providing food as well. Later, handyperson, gardening and home help services started. The overhead margin of around £5 per hour paid for DBS checks and administration; it was also hoped it would cross-subsidise general staff costs. But these services were not viable. Many 'handyperson' requests actually required more substantial builders' work and had to be refused. At £10 per hour for gardening, £15 for handyperson services and £13 to £14 for cleaners, all below the rates of agencies and even many self-employed individuals, it was difficult to recruit workers. This illustrates the difficulty of reconciling affordability for both client and worker in schemes of this kind.

The Circles projects have focused on recruiting over-50s to membership, so the only intergenerational contacts that members have are with volunteers – for example, the Rochdale drivers, although a few Rochdale members reported in the evaluation survey that they would like to see more younger people. North London Cares, founded in 2011 in Camden and Islington, had an explicitly intergenerational model, bringing seniors together with younger people in groups for parties, film shows, meals out, dance, cooking and book clubs (one of which the author ran from 2018 to 2020). Although younger people did most of the organising, with support of paid staff, both age groups were described as 'neighbours' to make them feel equal, neither group depending on a service from the other. A one-to-one visiting initiative was entitled 'Love My Neighbour', rather than a 'befriending scheme', to assert that the parties were equal friends, not provider and client. The main objective was mutual enjoyment of company and common interests, although younger neighbours sometimes did shopping, gardening or cooking for older ones. North London Cares also signposted people to National Health Service and council services they needed, and provided blankets, warm clothing and grants of up to £100 to people in fuel poverty.

Later, the 'Cares Family' started separate charitable companies in South London, East London, Manchester and Liverpool. Funding came from grants and donations. Members did some fundraising activity, but paid no formal subscription. Having brought together over 26,000 people, the 'Cares Family' ran out of money in the difficult fundraising environment following the COVID-19 pandemic, and closed in 2023.

In a consultant's evaluation of North London Cares and South London Cares (Renaisi, 2019), a survey of older 'neighbours' demonstrated considerable reduction in loneliness. But this had considerable cost; around £1,295 for each of 274 participants, although less if benefits for the 238 younger 'neighbours' were counted too. Many younger 'neighbours' were lonely newcomers to London. Intergenerational contacts may also have improved understanding of seniors' lives and needs. A younger 'neighbour' quoted in the evaluation report said: 'It helps me speak to older people and not be really prejudiced against older people. You learn more. I feel like I chat on the bus to older people more.'

The reduction in loneliness reduced formal care use in the first six months after joining the activities, although after 12 months, more care services were used than at the start. The evaluators attributed this to a decline in participants' health. However, the only way to be sure would have been to compare participants over time with a control group matched for age and initial health status.

All these staffed projects have very high costs. The task of expanding helpful friendships seems best achieved through informal contacts and existing voluntary organisations, as well as through developing neighbourhoods in ways conducive to neighbour interaction. More will be said about that in Chapter 7.

Conclusion

This chapter has explored the ways in which seniors can build and sustain supportive social relationships which address emotional as well as practical needs. Setting the scene, the work of Kartupelis emphasises the importance of compassion, empathy and friendship in formal care. Segal and the Care Collective echo this in relation to informal support as well, in their vision of the 'caring economy'. The Campsbourne Collective illustrated how households affected by caring and disability need to come together for sharing experiences and information, for mutual support and for defining their needs to present to formal services, individually and collectively.

Most important are the natural contacts through which people make friends. These are strongly affected by the kind of personal network they have; its scale, how dependent is it on family, how varied their contacts are in terms of the skills and strengths they bring and their links to sources of information and support. Intergenerational contacts and friendships are particularly valuable. The quality of the neighbourhood people live in – the sense of safety and whether it is easy to meet people – has considerable influence on personal networks. Housing and street design, the availability of community meeting places like pubs, parks, community centres and cafes, are all important.

Alleviating loneliness and isolation is a most important objective for preserving health and providing supportive contacts. It is not a panacea, since there are obviously many causes of ill health, and it should not be assumed that meeting many people necessarily helps to find *close* friends. Some people are more at risk of loneliness than others: lone parents; newcomers, especially migrants who speak a different language; and also people who are bogged down in their own health issues. Poor health and loneliness interact in a vicious circle.

Some community projects to address loneliness among seniors which have been taken as national models – the Cares Family, the Rochdale and other Circles – are shown to have rather high costs. Building a strategy against isolation on existing projects and clubs may be easier and cheaper than starting from scratch; the Leeds Neighbourhood Networks, described in Chapter 7, offer an example of this.

Informal support from beyond the family cannot deal with severe care needs – the bedroom and bathroom tasks require formal care or support from close relatives. But community support can help people to get out and socialise, maintain their home and garden, and help with smartphone and computer tasks.

Widening the caring circle

This chapter has illustrated the scale and type of needs that friends, neighbours and volunteers could address in a typical urban street.

The challenge is not large – perhaps 60–70 hours per week among over 300 non-disabled adults in a street of say 200 homes, or about two hours per person per month if say half of these 300 join in. The next chapter describes some solidarity projects through which this kind of support could be organised.

6

Solidarity projects: mutual aid, timebanks, community unions and volunteers

Introduction

This chapter describes the types of community project that might help to address the care deficit of coming years. It focuses on mutual aid, assessing its capacity to grow a culture of mutual support between neighbours, and to help build collective projects for supporting family carers and the growth of non-profit social enterprises. Mutual aid is broadly defined here; the examples described include the mutual aid groups (MAGs) of the COVID-19 pandemic period, timebanks and community unions. An example of traditional volunteering, the NHS Volunteer Responder scheme, is introduced by way of contrast, to show both its potential and its limitations.

MAGs and timebanks could support the growth of social enterprises, including micro-enterprises and care cooperatives, of the kind mentioned in Chapter 4. They can help to run collective services like day centres and lunch clubs. Like traditional volunteering, projects based on mutual aid principles have potential for augmenting the supply of informal care for individuals, but these principles are somewhat different from the traditional volunteering model and carry several advantages, as this chapter will describe. Timebanks may be considered a form of mutual aid, insofar as they offer exchanges of support between individuals. While this has been more prominent in their history in the United States, China and Japan, timebanks' main function in the UK has been to provide a volunteering opportunity which helps people build supportive personal friendship networks, alleviating isolation, and offering sociable exercise and a sense of purpose.

Some may wonder whether building the role of community projects in social care detracts from the need for expanded formal services. The growth of timebanks in the UK was encouraged by the 'Big Society' agenda of the Cameron government, with a view to reducing the demand for formal care. Like the other projects described here, they are examples of a 'strengths-based approach' to the care deficit. As Lunt (2019) points out, this approach walks a tightrope between a neoliberal role *replacing* state services and a more progressive one of enhancing them. The distinctive character of MAGs is that they lean towards the latter, often providing a channel for campaigning for *better* state services, while community unions are at the most political end of the four-type spectrum, and the NHS Volunteer Responders, following them, the least.

MAGs, timebanks and traditional volunteering all have potential for providing informal care to individuals. But their role is different from formal care; both are needed and they are actually complements to formal care rather than substitutes. As described in Chapter 5, there is a natural division of labour between intimate personal care, which is the bulk of what formal services do for seniors, and support with other aspects of life: home maintenance, internet access, information, socialising and mobility, which is the terrain of friends and volunteers. These forms of help address especially an early stage of age-related difficulties, meeting objectives of social inclusion and prevention of further decline.

A short history of mutual aid groups

MAGs arose throughout Europe during the COVID-19 pandemic (Sitrin and Colectiva Sembrar, 2020), and also to respond to natural disasters in the United States and elsewhere (Spade, 2020). Up to three million people in the UK are thought to have assisted neighbourhood MAGs (Tiratelli and Kaye, 2020). One survey of helpers found that on average they gave support on 17 occasions for 1.8 hours each time (Wein, 2020[1]). The number of groups has been estimated at 4,224 by the Office for National Statistics (2020b), or perhaps as many as 4,300 (O'Dwyer et al, 2021). The pandemic saw an extraordinary increase in volunteer activity. Alongside MAGs, the NHS Responder programme attracted 750,000 volunteers. Prior to the COVID-19 pandemic, organised volunteering provided only around 1 per cent of non-family social care in the UK (Cameron et al, 2020). The NHS Responder programme continues, but most MAGs in the UK became dormant or morphed into other forms as the pandemic retreated. By 2023, few remained to study as still-functioning groups, except where they were anchored to more permanent organisations like community centres or churches.

Frequently, MAGs have referred to their actions and values as 'solidarity'. Historically used in the trade union movement, this term is associated with unity in resistance: 'an injury to one is an injury to all' was the motto of the Industrial Workers of the World, founded in the United States in 1905. Just as trade unions seek to change employers' offers, 'solidarity' in the field of community organising implies commitment to seeking social change – in the offers of the state (central or local) or of social institutions more widely.

Solidarity implies that the community bond carries a sense of *collective agency for change*. This invites attempts to solve the problem that required support, by building new institutions, better community facilities or services. Solidarity does not necessarily involve reciprocation of all instances of help, nor an expectation of capacity to do so. But the bonds between community members will encourage people to give as well as receive if they can. Altruism, rather than reciprocity, features in some descriptions of solidarity offered by 'mutual' aid groups (Spade, 2020).

The Care Collective (Chatzidikis et al, 2020) sees MAGs as one potential foundation of a caring community, with precedents in the informal childcare collectives started by the women's movement in the 1970s, and in the history of the European

---

[1] A sample of 182 people who completed an online survey offered to MAGs registered on the national website; the information in the report is supplemented from several other sources.

cooperative movement. They envisage that mutual aid would sit alongside expanded and democratised state services, co-produced by the community: 'caring communities are democratic. They must extend localised engagement and governance through radical municipalism and cooperatives, and rebuild the public sector through expanding and insourcing its caring and welfare activities, rather than the outsourcing which accompanies privatisation' (Chatzidikis et al, 2020: 46).

The distinctive characteristics of mutual aid groups in the UK

Research on MAGs shows their distinctive and innovative role in developing communities' capacity for certain aspects of informal care (Tiratelli and Kaye, 2020; Benton and Power, 2021; Mayo, 2022). People came forward as neighbours helping each other, without distinctions between 'givers' and 'receivers'. They might shop for others when well, and be assisted if they themselves had to self-isolate. Needs were defined by what people said they wanted, rather than by any pre-defined model, leading to a flexible and open-ended array of forms of help. While the most typical tasks were shopping, collecting medicines and providing information, many others arose from requests, including pet care, gardening, friendly phone calls, cooked meal delivery, online yoga classes and quizzes (Benton and Power, 2021; Chevée, 2022). The informality of MAGs facilitated agility and speed of response to need, without assessment of who was 'deserving' or formal application processes. Some MAGs formed partnerships with charities, businesses and local government departments to deepen and sustain their work.

Although MAGs were often short-lived, they played a significant role in preventive support for seniors, helping them to go out, stay active and connected, reducing anxieties of those who live alone, doing DIY tasks – all important for healthy and sustained independent living. If revived at scale, they could also support intensive carers in similar ways and perhaps offer a few hours' respite care, lifts or social connections for those isolated by caring commitments.

Although by late 2023 most groups had left no trace on the national MAG listing site[2] except a Facebook page with closed

---

[2] UK National mutual aid groups website, https://covidmutualaid.org

membership, their legacy is assessed in several studies as a significant uplift in networking between neighbours (Wein, 2020; Mayo, 2022; Cocking et al, 2023). As lockdown continued, groups received fewer requests; possibly those needing support had found helpful neighbours and no longer required an intermediary. MAGs left behind a sense that people would get support again if they needed each other, providing reassurance and collective identity. Lasting achievements of MAGs, identified in a survey of Bristol groups (Jones et al, 2023), were mainly creation of social capital; increased frequency of neighbour connections and small acts of kindness, greater ease of forming support groups and organising community events. Likewise, in Wein's UK-wide survey, over half the participants said they would like to continue the same kinds of help after the pandemic. They showed higher levels of trust than in the general population.

The political role of mutual aid groups

Although most respondents to Wein's survey did not regard MAGs as political, 83 per cent of survey respondents were likely to take some political action, such as contacting a politician, signing a petition or attending a demonstration. Over half said the COVID-19 pandemic had changed how they thought about society.

The mutual aid movement internationally has often drawn inspiration from anarchist traditions (Kropotkin, 2009 [1902]; Preston and Firth, 2020; Spade, 2020). But the political role of British MAGs has not, overall, lived up to pro-anarchist ambitions of challenging social problems. By contrast, MAGs in New York were closely allied to struggles of homeless people and struggles against police brutality. Other international examples of MAGs pursued migrants' access to healthcare in Canada and land occupation to address food poverty in South Africa and the Lebanon. However, some UK groups did give support to Black Lives Matter or protested against politicians breaking lockdown rules (Kavada, 2022).

In the United States, mutual aid has been linked to long-term initiatives that have sought to support marginalised groups in contexts where they have been badly served, or not served at all, by state provision and by established charitable organisations. Within this strand are those started by the Black Panthers and Puerto Rican communities in the 1960s (Spade, 2020) and more recently by LGBTQIA+ and disabled Americans (Piepsna-Samarasinha, 2018). Mutual aiders, in these examples, see the state as neglectful, even antagonistic and manipulative of minorities, leading to an ambition for lasting collective support which is independent of the state while also challenging discrimination and neglect. Spade (2020) represents the anarchist strand of mutual aid as being very wary of 'co-optation' by state organs, generally preferring to operate independently to build capacity for system change. However, he relates how one American initiative, the Black Panthers' school breakfast programme, was eventually offered as a new state service.

Although MAGs in the United States have usually operated independently of state structures, Mayo (2022) argues for collaboration with local authorities. Although some councils were antagonistic to MAGs or ignored them, others provided support for COVID-19 MAGs in the form of coordination, information and training. Local authorities could also refer people needing help to MAGs, and vice versa. Participating in MAGs helped residents to develop a shared understanding of needs, a desire to press for better services, and an organisational basis for providing them if the state could not or would not do so. Thus they had potential to stimulate change in local authority services. Their starting point was discovering and listening to need rather than offering a pre-defined service. In this they differed from the traditional voluntary sector, which since the late 1990s has increasingly been led into sub-contracting for local authority services, for example, supporting people after hospital discharge, running day centres and providing mental health support. Such contractual arrangements, with tight boundaries of services framed with measurable outcomes to secure funding, tend to dampen innovation and responsiveness to newly discovered needs, as well as constraining political engagement.

The practical legacy of COVID-19 period mutual aid groups

The Care Collective sees MAGs as a potentially important organisational vehicle for actualising the 'commons of care'. Since few have survived, at least in their original form, is this merely a pipe dream? The author's attempts to survey those in one London borough resulted in a low response. By late 2021, they were mostly dormant. But several wider studies mentioned in this chapter indicate that MAGs have contributed to building neighbourly relationships, improving social networks and reciprocal capacity at local level, sowing the seeds of a future revival. Some have left a legacy of new activities, or important learnings, to the anchor organisations that gave birth to them. Three examples from one London borough illustrate different ways in which this has happened.

In April 2020, a MAG formed in the North London suburb of Haringey. It involved 600–700 terraced homes, mostly houses but some purpose-built maisonettes with gardens, both about three-quarters owner-occupied. Leaflets were distributed offering support to self-isolators; a WhatsApp group was established to help with shopping and medicine-fetching. In the beautiful spring weather of 2020, those on furlough developed an enthusiasm for gardening; swapping of plants became widespread through the WhatsApp group. People cooked more at home during lockdown, leading to exchanges of recipes and sometimes ingredients. Parents exchanged tips about children's activities and home tuition. This generated a huge uplift in social contacts across the neighbourhood. In July 2020, the WhatsApp group mobilised for a rally supporting Black Lives Matter; over 300 people attended a carefully distanced gathering in a park, called by residents of a nearby council estate that has a much higher Black population. By early 2024, the WhatsApp group survives as a valuable form of social connectivity. It carries borrowing requests for things like tools, garden equipment, visitors' parking permits, mislaid laptop chargers and printing facilities. People offer unwanted baby things, toys and furniture, reducing the rubbish stream. Money and clothes were collected for Ukrainian refugees and for victims of the Turkish earthquake in 2022. A monthly book club now meets in the pub. Volunteers have mobilised for weeding, planting and litter-picking in our local park, and are negotiating with the council for its improvement. The theme of helping vulnerable people was gradually replaced by general community messaging as lockdown eased. A lasting benefit of the group was neighbours' recommendations for trusted and economical builders and appliance repairers. Sadly, when some WhatsAppers offered to cook Christmas dinners for isolated seniors in 2020, none could be found – probably they existed but were not on WhatsApp, possibly among the one-third of seniors estimated still to have no smartphone (Age UK, 2024).

Another MAG in the same borough was formed by an established residents' association. Pandemic help with shopping morphed into a food bank, which continues in early 2024. Its additional services include citizen's advice sessions, a free clothing store, and occasional help with hospital transport, de-cluttering and gardening. Consistently with mutual aid principles, it requires no proof of 'deservingness' to receive food. Several other food banks in the borough share this feature, one loosely connected to a MAG in a very deprived council estate. Together they started a borough-wide food bank network which mobilised with local trade unions and around 20 community groups for a 'hunger march' in September 2023. This called for better social benefits, and action to address food poverty in the 'cost of living crisis' which followed the inflationary surge during the Ukraine war.

A third local example is the Campsbourne Community Collective, mentioned in Chapter 5. Residents there came together to push for improvements in local services around the time of the 2019 election. During the COVID-19 pandemic they formed a MAG with about 100 participants, doing food delivery with links to a local food bank, casework including supporting residents with benefit applications, and helping people obtain furniture from a charity recycling store. A befriending scheme was set up for residents in two sheltered housing schemes, using volunteers who already had DBS certificates for their usual jobs. Some members of another MAG, from private housing streets nearby, joined forces with these efforts. A long-term legacy was the community mapping project of local needs for public services, of which the 'care' part has been described in Chapter 5.

Timebanks: a variant of mutual aid?

Many of the features of MAGs have parallels in the timebanking movement, which forms a separate strand of reciprocal support for both individuals and collective community projects. Its history goes back to the 1970s in Japan, the 1980s in the United States, and the last 20–25 years in the UK. Timebanks often take on many of the features of mutual aid, though with some important differences, especially in the UK. Edgar Cahn, the founder of the American timebanking movement in the 1980s, saw timebanks as a way of mobilising seniors to help each other where formal care services are minimal. He regarded timebanks as a form of mutual aid, helping to fill the shortage of informal carers in the ageing society (Cahn and Gray, 2015). Pre-established timebanks have also provided emergency help, for example, in New Orleans in 2005, in Florida after a 1992 hurricane and in New Zealand after earthquakes in 2010 and 2011. Like MAGs, timebanks are often short-lived, but the more successful ones have endured several decades, accompanied by a voluminous literature.

Timebanks are distinct from MAGs in having a transactional element; the notion that members receive an hour of someone else's time and give an hour of their own in exchange. But, in practice, this feature is often dropped over time in favour of more fluid and unmeasured forms of reciprocity. In many other ways, they share key features with mutual aid; the concepts of co-production of activities by both providers and receivers; of equality of status between helpers and helped; an emphasis on sharing resources and developing community connections. Thus timebanking occupies a position between a distributional and a market logic; their transactional aspect operates with much less rigidity than a money exchange.

Timebank exchanges may be person to person, or from a member to the group, as in offering to cook lunch for a community meal. Service provision may be focused on support for carers or seniors, or can take the form of running group activities like a community centre, food growing project or youth group. The time-giver may earn an hour's worth of time from another member, or the right to participate in a group activity like a yoga session, a lunch, a computer lesson or an excursion. Sometimes rewards are donated by businesses or other organisations, enabling members to exchange time credits for shop or cafe discounts, tickets for the cinema, swimming pools or tourist attractions.

Dubb (2022) notes that while the transactional element distinguishes timebanks from MAGs, they share the notion that 'everyone has needs that should be met and that everyone has something to offer to help meet others' needs'. The transactional principle need not lead to a sense of debt by those who use more time than they give; timebankers often accumulate credits rather than 'spending' them, or donate credits to a common pool which can be given away (Clement et al, 2017). Thus several timebanks in the UK have come closer to the mutual aid model than the movement's founders envisaged.

Cahn and Gray (2021) report that in many timebanks, 'members understand that their time bank will never be able to "repay" them, but they donate hours of community service to the organization anyway ... the way that timebanks account for time credits is often intentionally loose'. They identify five core principles of timebanks which are similar to those of mutual aid:

1. An asset perspective – everyone has something to contribute.
2. Redefining what we value as work – volunteering counts as 'work'.
3. Reciprocity, or a 'pay-it-forward' ethos.
4. Interdependence and community building.
5. Mutual accountability and respect.

Another similarity is the emphasis on co-production by service users, an important aspect of the timebank model (Cahn and Gray, 2011) which it shares with the values of MAGs. For example, the Hull and East Riding Timebank includes in its mission statement: 'Redefine the nature of work and consumption by using the power of our mutual aid networks to inspire, train and support people to co-create new regenerative, rewarding and dignified livelihoods through social enterprises and co-operatives.'[3] Where all involved in offering or receiving services help to shape the project, this can improve quality of services and activities, and creates a collective drive to seek more resources where needed.

---

[3] Hull and East Riding Timebank, https://www.timebankhullandeastriding.co.uk/blank-1

The principle of reciprocity raises the question: how can people benefit who have nothing to offer, either because of their health status or because of heavy caring commitments? However, the capacity of older seniors, even housebound people, to reciprocate may be under-estimated. It can include important forms of peer support on health issues, through which substantially age-impaired people have found opportunities to reciprocate support, gaining self-esteem and social contacts (Boneham and Sixsmith, 2006; NAPA, 2012, cited in Gray and Worlledge, 2018). Pet feeding, receiving deliveries, cooking, clothing repair, pot-plant care, knitting and craft work offer other possibilities for people with limited mobility or strength. Appendix C provides several examples of mutual aid between neighbours in sheltered housing schemes for seniors.

Timebanks and the state: a problematic relationship

Timebanks have had a very different relationship to the state from MAGs. Their promotion, as part of the coalition government's 'Big Society' perspective, gave rise to a mushrooming of start-ups around 2011–14, often with substantial public funding. Drawing on the Blair government's ideas of the 'Third Way' (Blair, 1998), Cameron's government sought to sub-contract some public sector tasks to low-cost, voluntary sector sub-contractors (Espiet-Kilty, 2016). It drew voluntary organisations into contracts, which restricted lobbying and campaigning, denying voice and innovative capacity (Cushman and Millbourne, 2015). Wilson (2015) cautions against timebanks being coopted into a 'Big Society' model which aims to *reduce* social service costs. Cameron's 'Big Society' sought to create community organisations to replace some formal services, or at least create social capital from which informal care would expand to allow their shrinkage. However, the value of timebanks in practice has not been to generate person-to-person help; this has only been achieved on a small scale in the UK and at very high costs. Rather, their achievements have been in alleviating isolation, helping people to make social contacts through volunteering and social events.

The Cameron government, seeking to mobilise volunteers to trim the welfare state's bills, drew inspiration from Japanese timebanks. Hayashi (2012), drawing on Japanese experience, saw timebanks as contributing to the 'Big Society' agenda. However, the history of timebanking in Japan itself was more about growing new services, to supplement scarce formal services for seniors, than replacing them or reducing their costs. Timebanking in the 1990s was used to address a care deficit of emergency proportions; under-developed social services had left the ageing Japanese society with enormous unmet needs and unsustainable burdens for family carers. When long-term care insurance, introduced in 2000, provided more resources for formal care, timebanking retreated in scale.

The dual role of timebanks: more social contacts than practical support

Most of the longer-lived UK timebanks started with the goal of person-to-person support, but gradually focused more on individual-to-project support. Their main value is in combating loneliness and sustaining community projects that help to do that. The Blair government promoted them to generate social capital in deprived neighbourhoods as part of the 'Third Way' communitarian approach to developing socially cohesive communities, in which people would help each other, reducing dependence on the state as well as loneliness. This approach could be considered a route to a 'smaller state', particularly when linked to the 'Big Society' ambitions of the succeeding Conservative government. But it was also a vehicle for useful thinking about the importance of social relationships for seniors, and the contexts in which they could flourish and be sustained: 'Everyone, including older people, has the right to participate and continue throughout their lives having meaningful relationships and roles. Older people's vital role and responsibility to help build social capital will become ever more apparent as our society ages' (Social Exclusion Unit, 2006: 8).

Generally, timebanks in the UK have contributed more to building personal networks and supporting community centres, or other collective projects like community gardens, than they have generated services to individuals. There are good reasons for this. Risk assessment, safeguarding and supervision of person-to-person help are very time-consuming tasks requiring a paid worker, which creates dependence on external salary funding (Naughton-Doe et al, 2021). At the extreme, this leads to costs of person-to-person help per hour which can be as high as for paid workers; for example, in Cambridgeshire villages it varied between £17 and £27 per hour (Cambridge Centre for Housing and Planning Research, 2014). Thus many timebanks do not last beyond three years, frequently the timespan of their initial grant. At most, 150 were operating in Great Britain by around 2019, reduced from a peak of around 3,000 in 2012–15 (Cahn and Gray, 2015; Spinelli et al, 2019).

Time-givers are sometimes highly vulnerable people, resulting in a heavy load for the worker supporting and supervising them. Thus a trade-off may exist between social integration of members, and providing a desired volume of reliable services. To avoid the difficulty of supervision in one-to-one settings, services for individuals are often replaced by group activities, and credits are offered for helping with them to encourage participation. These credits may be spent on other activity sessions, including 'treats' donated by businesses such as discounts or gym sessions. Many timebanks use the concept of time exchange to attract people into co-production and co-organising of social events and groups such as shared meals, community gardening, film nights, knitting and sewing circles. In the example of the Hull and East Riding Timebank, founded in 2012,[4] these events, rather than services to individual non-members, are the main focus. Likewise, Fair Shares in Gloucestershire, now 25 years old, has dropped the accounting of time given and received, and just engages participants in creating activities for each other like gardening, cooking, hobby sessions and trips so that they can feel included and make friends. Rushey Green, a London timebank, started in a doctor's surgery over two decades ago. Many timebank members are recruited through 'social prescribing' to encourage them to socialise and keep active. They benefit from the friendship and support of other members, with whom they can attend group social activities organised by the timebank, including community

---

[4] Hull and East Riding Timebank, https://www.timebankhullandeastriding.co.uk/blank-1

gardening, tea and chat sessions, a choir, making jewellery and toys for fundraising sales, 'bring and fix' sessions for mutual help with repairing clothes and domestic items. In 2016–17, Rushey Green left the doctor's surgery and developed a large partnership of voluntary organisations, Lewisham Local,[5] which has about 20 projects offering a wide variety of volunteering opportunities and social events. Before the COVID-19 pandemic, when many activities were suspended, DIY tasks and gardening for seniors were offered between timebank members. Rather than visiting homes as before, the focus is now on activities which take place in the Lewisham Local centre.

Delivery of interpersonal services through timebanking has been better developed in Japan, the United States and in China than in Britain. Chinese timebanking has been widely used to provide informal care for seniors with distant or few relatives. Linked schemes spread over several provinces enable credits earned in one region to be used in another, for a far-away relative to 'buy' support from their local scheme[6] – a huge advantage in a society where migration often separates generations. Most Chinese timegivers are recently retired people, often supporting older ones. They help with practical tasks but generally not intimate care. A rare exception is in the city of Nanjing, where social work trainees support professionals in tasks of 'meal assistance, bath assistance, cleaning assistance, emergency assistance, and medical support' (Wang, 2023).

In the United States, timebanks have developed to fill needs which are largely unmet by public services, since formal care there depends very heavily on private purchases from care agencies. Ryan-Collins et al (2008) describe a New York scheme in which residents exchanged services like shopping, cooking, escorting to medical appointments, computer support and housework. Seventy per cent of members were over 50 and two-fifths lived alone. Exchanging services helped them extend their support networks and feel assured of help when they needed it. Another American example is 'Partners in Care' in Maryland (Cahn and

---

[5] Lewisham Local, https://www.lewishamlocal.com/our-projects/
[6] As described by Professor Xiaoying Wang in a webinar organised by Timebanking UK in September 2023.

Gray, 2015). Started as a timebank, it is now partly a 'volunteer exchange' with no recording of hours given or received, and also provides non-profit services for cash. The volunteer exchanges include telephone befriending, peer support groups for veterans and visually impaired people, lifts, computer support, and DIY tasks including minor home adaptations like grab rails.[7]

Some timebanks which do offer person-to-person support enable members to 'bank' time credits over a long period, so they can build up credits when active and use them when they are sick. This could be attractive to seniors worried about how to manage during sickness. Examples of it are found in China (Wang, 2023) and Japan (Singh, 2017), and an American scheme, Give&Take Care (Spinelli et al, 2019). An attempt to replicate Give&Take Care in the UK was launched in 2015. By 2018, it was operating in Wokingham, Slough, Rochdale and Leicester,[8] charging a £5 annual membership fee and £1 per hour for administrative costs to people referred by GPs or social agencies to receive services. Time-givers, often seniors themselves, offered befriending, shopping, lifts to medical appointments, help with cleaning and paperwork, gardening, support in day centres and respite for family carers. Although still registered as a Community Interest Company, Give&Take Care appears no longer to be active.

Fair Shares also tried a 'credit saving' facility (Boyle and Bird, 2014). Time-givers could build up credit by providing help, then call on others for two weeks' support during a later period of illness. This feature no longer exists as a distinct 'offer' of membership, but its current time-broker (spoken to by the author in 2024) says that members often do develop friendships in which this kind of delayed reciprocity can occur without transactional accounting.

These examples show how timebanking has some potential for mutual support between individuals, particularly for isolated seniors or for people seeking to exchange efforts to secure informal help for relatives living in another area. However, the cost of safeguarding and organisational overheads can be very high.

---

[7] https://partnersincare.org/service-exchange/
[8] Exposure Press blog, 20 April 2020, https://exposure.press/givetakecare-the-community-looking-after-itself/

Community unions

The community union, ACORN, is a strand of mutual aid with a particularly strong political thrust. Started in the United States in 1970, ACORN campaigned for a living wage and attempted to create a new trade union for unorganised and precarious workers. Among its successes were securing smaller school classes and other educational improvements, affordable housing for homeless people in several cities, and reducing discrimination in mortgage lending. In New Orleans, after Hurricane Katrina in 2005, ACORN supported poor, mainly Black, communities against their neighbourhoods being re-developed for the use of higher-income groups. Its volunteers helped clean and re-build flood-damaged homes. ACORN developed international offshoots in several other countries before the American organisation closed in 2010 following an intense political campaign against it which involved some findings of fraudulent voter registration and financial irregularity (Beck and Purcell, 2013). Its surviving legacy was the international organisation, active in 11 countries, including Canada, Kenya and India.

ACORN set up in Bristol in 2014, and by early 2024 had developed branches in 24 other areas of England[9] with differently named groups in Scotland (Living Rent) and Northern Ireland (Community Action Tenants Union). It aims to marshal community support for those who need others to help them combat injustice. ACORN belongs to the category of a mutual aid organisation rather than a campaigning group because of its strong focus on individual casework, both as an end in itself and as a learning process. Typically ACORN interventions begin by finding out about individuals' problems, usually through house-to-house surveys. It presses their case with the landlord or service providers, then identifies others who have similar problems, leading where possible to negotiations with the company or local authority to secure resolution for all of them. Sometimes the solution aims for national legislation, like ACORN's current

---

[9] ACORN, https://www.acorntheunion.org.uk/; personal communication from ACORN national office; *Morning Star*, 18 February 2019, 'ACORN UK; Taking what's ours'.

support for the Renters' Reform Bill. ACORN's approaches to negotiate are often backed by direct action in the form of pickets or blockades, especially when defending tenants against eviction. In England, it has focused particularly on housing issues, also including repairs, heating and letting agents' practices, ACORN has secured better bus services in Oxfordshire, and persuaded Bristol Council to abandon plans to scrap its council tax reduction scheme. In Leeds, they took a giant cardboard skip to a councillor's 'surgery' to negotiate better rubbish collections and litter removal.

Among issues of concern to seniors, ACORN has campaigned to re-open closed public toilets in Bristol, Brighton and Newcastle. It has also taken action to support residents in sheltered housing, for example winning concessions for residents who were in dispute with their Brighton landlord over food services and management charges. In Swindon, withdrawal of full-time 'wardens' from several sheltered housing schemes left residents feeling unsafe and unsupported; nine months of lobbying the council won a promise of three new full-time warden posts.

ACORN exhibits an important principle of mutual aid; people who don't themselves experience a problem taking collective action for those who do, by trying to find long-term solutions through changes in policy and practice of those in authority. The financial model is also a promising one; ACORN members, now numbering over 10,000 in the UK, pay monthly dues like a conventional trade union. Together with donations from non-members and external funding, this has enabled the organisation to employ paid organisers and like its parent organisation did in the United States, to build up substantial assets for expansion.

The NHS Volunteer Responder programme

Launched by the NHS in March 2020 with its organising partner, the Royal Voluntary Service (RVS), this programme helped people who were affected by the COVID-19 pandemic by delivering food and medicines, transporting patients or equipment, and helpful phone calls to reassure people or provide information. Over 750,000 people came forward, although some were not accepted onto the programme after vetting, and others dropped out. Thus only around 436,000 actually put themselves 'on duty' through the phone app that allocated tasks (Dolan et al, 2021). However, the national system could barely cope with the number of volunteers and almost two-fifths had not been allocated any task by August 2020. Some modifications were made to the phone app to avoid this – for example, if the response needed was merely a phone call, spreading the request for someone to make it over a wider geographical area. Nonetheless, one-fifth of volunteers only ever completed one task during three to four months, and only half did five or more tasks.

In autumn 2020, the NHS and RVS surveyed over 12,000 of the Volunteer Responders (NHS with Royal Voluntary Service, 2020). They found that one-fifth were volunteering for the first time when they joined the programme during the pandemic. Over two-thirds were interested in continuing, although another survey in 2022 found that only 45 per cent had actually done so (NHS, 2023). This suggests a major upsurge in volunteering following the pandemic – over 1 per cent of the national total of adults had become newly engaged. The question is how it might best be utilised in the longer term.

The 2022 survey found that volunteers wanted more opportunity to share experiences and participate in planning future developments. By seeking further feedback through webinars, phone calls and social media, the organisers found that volunteers were interested in providing a wider range of services.

A separate survey of patients showed that one-third had contacted the responder service themselves, or had a friend or relative do so. However, the majority were referred through doctors, hospitals or local authority staff. Most were seniors, and were very satisfied with the service, but some wanted more sustained contact with volunteers with more variety and control about the kind of tasks they could ask for. RVS then contacted 6,000 clients to find out what support they needed. More 'bespoke' services are now being planned for people with greater needs (NHS with Royal Voluntary Service, 2021).

The experience of the NHS responders illustrates the rigidity of a very large national programme. Its continuation has focused on getting people to offer a limited range of pre-specified tasks, centrally organised through a phone app: shopping, fetching medicine, and 'check in and chat' by a phone call to 'vulnerable' and lonely people. In June 2023, the Department of Health and Social Care announced that the Volunteer Responder programme would expand into social care.[10] The aim was to help people being discharged from hospital and enable them to be discharged sooner. 'Check in and chat plus' now provides a phone call up to three times a week for six weeks. A survey of health and other professionals who had referred people to the programme (NHS with Royal Voluntary Service, 2021) found that almost two-thirds of referrals requested phone calls, with a quarter of these being for the six-week arrangement. Hopefully the programme will develop greater variety and flexibility of tasks in future, building on the feedback from clients and volunteers. The flexibility and *unboundaried* character of what MAGs provided contrasts with the narrow, fixed remit of the NHS programme so far.

Mutual aid projects in the future of solidarity

Timebanks and MAGs have a very different financial and leadership basis, and tend to attract different types of people. Starting a MAG required leadership and initiative, often without funding, paid workers or premises, although some were based on an existing community centre or church. Their start-up involved bringing neighbours together, setting up a new WhatsApp or a Facebook group, producing leaflets, sourcing free food and transport, organising people to canvass a street to find who needed support and who could give it. But unless they morphed into other more permanent forms of community action, MAGs did not need to address long-term sustainability and its frequent requirements of funding, insurance and a physical base. Timebanks, on the other hand, have mainly had start-up funding for a paid development worker, often an 'anchor' organisation which provided premises and a focal point for activity and recruitment. With their emphasis on building social capital, timebanks offer isolated people a menu of pre-defined activities within an established, funded framework. Significantly, a survey of around 850 MAG members found

---

[10] Press release from Department of Health and Social Care, 7 June 2023, https://www.gov.uk/government/news/successful-nhs-programme-to-recruit-care-volunteers

that they were predominantly middle class, from communities that were older, happier and wealthier than average (O'Dwyer et al, 2021). MAGs formed more frequently in higher-income areas with a relatively large proportion of university graduates (Felici, 2020). Whereas MAGs in the pandemic were founded by people who *had* connections, had social capital, timebanks have attracted people who wanted to *make* connections. Thus although timebanks share many foundational principles with MAGs, differences are apparent in the underlying social networks of the membership, the kind of people they have attracted and their costs.

Some local models for development of community solidarity

Suffolk and Essex have shown how new forms of non-profit care of the kinds mentioned in Chapter 4 can be built on the back of volunteering and mutual aid during the COVID-19 pandemic. They offer important examples of developing volunteering and micro-enterprise in rural areas. The legacy of helping the community during the pandemic has helped micro-enterprise development; an Essex County Council assessment of the provider market states that 'COVID introduced many new people to the social care sector through volunteering and raised awareness, and this has encouraged some people to set up their own business offering support to others in their community'.[11] During the pandemic, the county council brought together a partnership of voluntary organisations to support the community through the emergency, under the title the Essex Wellbeing Service. Many volunteers who joined it continue to offer support to others through a phone app which is currently being trialled in Basildon. Volunteers are also recruited through local Facebook groups.[12]

---

[11] Essex County Council Provider Hub, *Community Microenterprises*, https://www.essexproviderhub.org/the-essex-market/market-position-statement/market-enablers/community-micro-enterprises/

[12] Essex County Council, *Tribe Case Study*, https://tribeproject.org/static/cases/Tribe_CaseStudy_Essex.pdf

In 2019, Suffolk and Essex county councils came together in a new drive to support development of micro-enterprises, linking them to volunteers and voluntary organisations. This was seen as an important aspect of 'personalisation' of care, encouraging and supporting people to take up personal budgets as well as link them to their communities and develop personal contacts. The project encouraged former volunteers and people who had been family carers to start micro-enterprises. Essex commissioned a micro-enterprise development organisation, the Tribe Project CIC, to pilot a mobile phone app which links potential users of services to volunteer groups, paid providers, social activities and events. Tribe is also mapping service provision to see where there are geographical gaps, and offering training to existing providers to help fill those gaps.

Seeing a potential and promising transition from volunteering to providing part-time services for pay, Essex offered organisational development support for people to start micro-enterprises. Tribe provides DBS checks, training and a 'gateway' to link new enterprises to clients. The local Council for Voluntary Service offers free help with setting up a Community Interest Company or a charity. Micro-enterprises often adopt one of these legal forms, although they may alternatively be sole traders, partnerships or ordinary companies.

Based on previous experience, Tribe expects that micro-enterprise can achieve a saving of one third in the cost of homecare, and raise pay by 36 per cent compared to 2019 levels. By March 2023, Essex had 76 micro-enterprises, with over 50 in development. The average hourly cost of homecare was £17.50, much less than commercial agencies.

From 2022, Suffolk County Council developed a large network of micro-enterprises to serve villages and small towns, one of several dozen micro-enterprise projects run by Community Catalysts in different parts of England. Suffolk's directory of 70 micro-enterprises offers homecare and day services, and in some cases home helps.[13] This micro-enterprise initiative built on the legacy of a rich history of volunteer support, formerly provided

---

[13] Community Catalysts, https://www.communitycatalysts.co.uk/smallgoodstuff/directory

at four sites in the county by the national charity, Age UK, which sadly closed in 2020 due to a sudden drop in public sector funding during the pandemic. According to Suffolk Age UK's final annual report, over 240 volunteers provided several thousand hours of support per year to around one senior in 200 across the county. Their services included housework, companionship and support with getting out and about, information or advice and telephone befriending. Much of this kind of work is now offered by micro-enterprises.

Conclusion

The examples presented here suggest that a revival of mutual aid groups, possibly hybridised in some instances with timebanks or non-profit care providers, could play a significant role in sustaining the volume of informal care that is needed.

However, it is important to bear in mind the appropriate 'division of labour' between formal services and help from outside the family. As noted in Chapter 5 and Appendix B, friends and neighbours very rarely cross the bedroom door; bedroom and bathroom tasks are best left to intimates or paid care workers. Where support is arranged through an organisation, safeguarding policies and DBS checks need to be in place, although MAGs during the pandemic emergency frequently did without. But organisational formalities should not create an artificial boundary between the activities the volunteer is sent to do and additional requests from the person visited that they may wish to accept. Volunteers may develop into friends; in the timebank world this is indeed one objective, and often it happens naturally within mutual aid structures.

Mutual aid groups, volunteer organisations and informal neighbourly help can give important support for activities which the formal care system rarely has the resources to offer seniors enough time for – shopping, non-routine cleaning tasks, cooking, helping people go out and about, support with IT and paperwork. While formal support services for people with dementia, learning disabilities or neuro-diversity may extend more to these areas, many seniors will find the bulk of these tasks falls outside their care plan. Non-relatives can provide vital help with safety-critical tasks, like removing trip hazards in carpeting, shifting heavy furniture or stepladder jobs. Help with garden maintenance or cooking the occasional special meal, or support with digital devices, may make considerable difference to someone's quality of life. Perhaps above all, the need for friendship, mobility support and inclusion in events outside the home is a crucial one that neither the homecare worker nor a weekly visit or phone call from a befriending scheme can adequately meet.

Volunteer support can take two forms: helping individuals directly, or helping collective projects to support carers and people with care needs. Collective projects may include day centres, lunch clubs or community centres that offer meeting places and activities, organised social activities in supported housing schemes, or advice centres. Day centres are important for carers as well as their users, since they offer respite which gives carers time on their own and may support them to maintain part-time employment. But as mentioned in Chapter 1, many have been lost during the decade of austerity. Lunch clubs and advice services have also declined in recent years since community centres have been hit by a shortage of council funding. A study of social enterprises – defined broadly by its authors as Community Interest Companies – in three English local authorities found that day services were their main contribution to the social care landscape, and that one-third of these enterprises had volunteers or were even run by them (Hall and Alexander, 2023).

Mutual aid projects and timebanks could help to reinforce these and other facilities that have been emasculated in the years of austerity. Sheltered housing schemes are without the full-time managers they once enjoyed, who had more time to befriend residents and organise social activities for them. Except where paid activity organisers are employed, collective activities often survive on the shoulders of a small, over-stretched group of volunteers, with considerable attrition as they age (Gray and Worlledge, 2018). Many day centres have survived only with reduced funding. Budget cuts in recent years have left many community centres almost bereft of paid staff, with reduced offerings of clubs and classes. The 'take and give' principle involved in timebanking may help to establish a sense of shared responsibility for activities which can no longer depend on paid staff, making people aware of the many tasks to be covered in organising events and caretaking of the venue. It could help to avoid dependence on a few volunteers, often themselves ageing, and give people a voice and a sense of ownership of precious community facilities.

During the pandemic emergency, MAGs tended to operate without public or charitable funding because they could often dispense with many formalities, and individual generosity provided for expenses of publicity and phone calls for a temporary period. For any project delivering individual person-to-person services in 'normal' circumstances, risk assessment and safeguarding are time-consuming tasks requiring a paid worker. This creates dependence on external salary funding. Spinelli et al (2019) argue this is why many timebanks do not last beyond three years, often the timespan of their start-up grant. Longer-term public or charitable funding is needed for such projects to continue, since they are unlikely to break even just from member subscriptions, selling services and/or fundraising activities. Apart from staff, other costs include software, phone and travel expenses, publicity, criminal record checks and training. Office space can often be obtained through another organisation, such as council offices, community centres, village halls and traditional voluntary service hubs. 'Anchor organisations' like these can provide a physical base and a flow of people from whom participants can be recruited.

With these practical issues in mind, the history of both MAGs and timebanks suggests several ways in which community solidarity in general could augment informal care or maintain seniors' health and independence. However, to approach the ambitions of the Care Collective for rebuilding and democratising the public sector, an additional political thrust is needed: solidarity for change. This is crucial to ensure that 'widening the circle' of care activism through community development does not collapse into the 'Big Society' model with unpaid community labour attempting to address the bulk of the care deficit.

Community unionism occupies a space between conventional trade unions and mutual aid groups. It has a strong political thrust for change, and has contributed to resolving local instances of injustice, especially about housing issues, in many English cities. It is distinctive in drawing funds for paid organisers from membership dues, without dependence on grant funding or public service contracts. There seem to be no recorded instances of action on specifically social care issues, but the potential may be there.

All these strands of activism are different in many ways from the traditional volunteering model of the NHS Volunteer Responders. However, that initiative shows how the pandemic has led to a considerable rise of interest in volunteering, with participants eager to move away from the limited array of tasks put forward by the scheme managers and develop more varied, flexible connections with the communities they wish to support.

What would it take to establish a 'commons of care' in which isolated seniors and disabled people, and their carers, can expect to share non-intimate tasks as a collective responsibility? There is a need to grow long-term supportive organisations which could offer, through membership groups and neighbourly support, the kind of services that MAGs and timebanks have undertaken. It also requires effective popular pressure to preserve and expand the core of professional formal care services, especially for personal care, which is outwith the scope of informal care except among close relatives, who may often be stressed. Such political pressure requires foregrounding of the eldercare and disability support agenda, giving an adequate voice to those who need support. Important related goals are helping them and their carers to build personal networks, to be respected and included, and face as few physical and social barriers as possible in daily living. Achievement of these goals can help to improve health and quality of life. This could somewhat reduce the need for care, whether paid or unpaid. The next chapter explores further how this could be done.

7

Reducing the need for care

Introduction

Health preservation strategies, to keep people well and independent for longer, are crucial to reduce the need for care and support. More people are surviving to their late 80s and beyond, but not surviving in good health. Around 27 per cent of those receiving social care across the life-span are over 85, and 11 per cent 75–84.[1] As mentioned in Chapter 3, the likely cost of health and care services is substantially affected by the age at which impairments of older age begin.

Fortunately the incidence of difficulties with activities of daily living (ADLs) among seniors has fallen between 2011 and 2021, from 31.3 per cent to 26 per cent.[2] But this might not continue, since arthritis,[3] diabetes[4] and dementia[5] are all rising rapidly. Healthy life expectancy at birth has been falling since 2006–8, more for women than for men (Centre for Ageing Better, 2022). Those who were already 65 just before the COVID-19 pandemic

---

[1] Statistica, 2022/23, https://www.statista.com/statistics/1233394/distribution-of-care-recipient-by-age-in-the-united-kingdom/
[2] HSE 2011 and 2018, author's analysis, and published report for 2021.
[3] https://www.keele.ac.uk/about/news/2022/october/proportion-adults/arthritis-diagnosis-increased.php
[4] Diabetes UK, 2023, https://www.diabetes.org.uk/about-us/about-the-charity/our-strategy/statistics
[5] Alzheimer's Research UK, 2024, https://dementiastatistics.org/about-dementia/prevalence-and-incidence/

could expect to live 9.8 to 9.9 more years disability-free, followed by 8.9 years with some disability. A key concern of public health services, in which the community can play an important role, is therefore extending healthy life expectancy and reducing prevalence of long-term conditions from middle age onwards.

People with early-stage or minor impairments could be helped a lot by preventive measures through the kind of support the community can give. If you have a painful arthritic knee, support with heavy shopping, or company for a gentle walk, may stop you getting worse. If you lack strength and energy for house jobs, help with fixing a loose handrail or tidying high cupboards may prevent a fall. Diabetes, heart disease or arthritis can be aggravated by cold; draught-proofing, advice about home insulation and avoiding fuel poverty is something many volunteer projects and friends can help with. Social inclusion of people with impairments, whatever their age, enabling them to minimise the impact of their difficulties on going out, meeting people and leisure pursuits, is also very important just to maximise their quality of life.

Improving the quality of life includes, in the words of the Chief Medical Officer for Health: 'Things which can be done to adapt the environment to allow an individual with a set amount of disability in older age to live as independent and enjoyable a life as possible … [this] includes issues around urban planning, building design, social care and aids to independent living' (Whitty, 2023, p 1). While a valuable reminder that social care should not be the neglected little sister of health services, this statement also emphasises the importance of other social policies in helping people manage impairments.

Ways of addressing preventive health objectives to be discussed in this chapter include:

- advice about healthier lifestyles;
- reducing poverty;
- addressing loneliness and isolation;
- better housing, including sheltered housing, extra-care housing and home adaptations;
- reducing the impact of long-term conditions and age-related impairments through change in social and physical environments.

A useful framework for developing such actions is 'age-friendly communities', a policy agenda developed by the World Health Organization which has been adopted by 83 local authorities across the UK, including Manchester, Leeds, seven London boroughs, Brighton, North Norfolk and the Isle of Wight. Many similar approaches have been adopted by councils that have not formally declared themselves to be 'age-friendly communities', including several rural areas (Whitty, 2023), which often have relatively high proportions of seniors in their populations. Developed by the World Health Organization (WHO, 2024) and promoted in the UK by the Centre for Ageing Better,[6] the age-friendly communities agenda contains eight 'domains' for policies to improve seniors' quality of life: outdoor spaces and buildings; transport; housing; social participation, respect and social inclusion; civic participation and employment; communication and information; community support; and health services. By improving health and reducing barriers to everyday living for age-affected people, policies across these areas can help reduce the need for eldercare, formal or informal. Many such measures can help younger disabled people and carers too. Also important is reducing air pollution, thought to cause thousands of deaths and cases of serious heart and lung conditions in the UK every year.

The right social and physical environment can help people to meet, know and trust each other, remaining engaged with their communities. This reduces the risk of loneliness and of physical and mental inactivity. Design of housing, of streets and gardens, adequacy and quality of public transport and community facilities (shops, parks, cafes and community centres) are all important to help people meet others and preserve their capacity for independence. These are aspects of neighbourhood quality, mentioned in Chapter 5 as a key factor in developing personal support networks.

Community centres need to be preserved as a vital base for such services and as places for intergenerational contact. Younger people can provide valuable support to social activities in sheltered housing.[7] Appreciation of seniors' views and empathy with them,

---

[6] Centre for Ageing Better, https://www.ageing-better.org.uk
[7] Abbeyfield Housing blog, https://www.abbeyfield.com/blog/exploring-the-benefits-of-intergenerational-activities/

gained through intergenerational contacts, is also an important foundation for widening the support circle, and raising the priority of formal care on the political agenda.

Through local examples of good practice in maximising social inclusion and reducing the need for care, often based on 'age-friendly communities' strategies, this chapter illustrates how community solidarity and the 'third sector' have important potential roles to play in improving the quality of life and keeping down the rising cost of formal care. This requires coordination of paid and unpaid care for the individual and at neighbourhood level. The chapter ends with some thoughts about how this could be achieved in a 'caring neighbourhood' of the future.

Policies for 'age-friendly communities': better places, better health, less need for care

The 'age-friendly communities' framework brings the eight domains together in a holistic way which gives space to co-production of policies with seniors themselves. Policies of this kind do not depend on local state action alone. The council is usually the leader of a partnership of local public sector actors with the voluntary sector; but sometimes the voluntary sector leads, as in the example of Age UK in Barnet, North London.[8]

Greater Manchester offers an important example of holistic age-friendly policies. The city launched its Age Friendly City strategy in 2016,[9] aiming to become a global centre of excellence for policies on ageing. It features a strong emphasis on early help and preventive health measures as ways to reduce care demand. This includes a wide offer of social activities and exercise, and a falls prevention programme. Carers' services include helping people access available cash benefits, an emergency support fund and a plan to expand respite care.

Through consultative workshops with older residents, Manchester has developed plans for improving pavements,

---

[8] https://www.barnet.gov.uk/news/plan-make-barnet-age-friendly-borough-officially-launched

[9] https://www.greatermanchester-ca.gov.uk/media/1166/gm_ageing_strategy.pdf

pedestrian crossings, bus stops, bus design, public seating and toilets (Musselwhite, 2018). Many urban features can be designed to make public spaces more accessible to age-affected and mobility-impaired people, helping them to experience fewer physical barriers to everyday living. Plentiful public toilets are very important, as are seats and resting places in parks and shopping centres, easy parking for mobility-impaired people and carers, lifts and entrance ramps at public buildings and stations.

Residents' lobbying plays a key role in pressing for age-friendly and disability-friendly services. An example is the London Loos Campaign,[10] which demands that each London borough establish a toilet strategy for improving the number and quality of public toilets. The growing interest in co-production in local government services offers opportunities for a citizen's voice about service development.

An age-friendly transport strategy has been recognised as important in helping seniors to keep active and travel without excessive dependence on taxis. Manchester, like the Isle of Wight, introduced training of bus drivers to be aware of disabled or age-affected people's needs.[11] Subsidised door-to-door transport, with helpful drivers for those with mobility issues, is important for health appointments and for access to seniors' social groups, lunch clubs or day centre services.

Reducing isolation and loneliness

Increasingly, health and care professionals are concerned to reduce isolation and loneliness in the hope of maintaining health and reducing the need for formal care.

As mentioned in Chapter 5, the importance of community projects to address isolation has been recognised by the practice of 'social prescribing', increasingly used by the National Health Service to address the downward spiral of isolation and ill health by referring people to exercise, gardening, art and music sessions, and other social activities within the community. In addition,

---

[10] Age UK website on 'London Loos' campaign, 2022 to 2024, https://www.ageuk.org.uk/london/projects-campaigns/out-and-about/london-loos/
[11] Centre for Ageing Better, https://ageing-better.org.uk/

the National Academy of Social Prescribing's evidence review (Sabey et al, 2022) shows positive health benefits under several headings which frequently involve voluntary sector provision. These include tackling food insecurity through lunch clubs and heathy cooking sessions, supporting digital inclusion to improve access to health and care services and social connectivity, and addressing fuel poverty through managing energy consumption and choosing suitable supplier contracts.

Core funding is needed for community centres and voluntary sector support to provide the capacity for these activities. Such investment requires a long-term coordinated approach to the desired outcomes across community, care and health budgets.

Digital exclusion

Digital exclusion, which affects a high proportion of seniors, needs to be tackled as a barrier to many aspects of life: accessing medical services, council and benefits services, online shopping, entertainment, neighbourhood WhatsApp and Facebook groups, keeping in touch with distant friends and relatives. Internet use will always be difficult for those who feel they are too old to learn or remember computer and smartphone procedures. (Hyacinth, in Appendix C, exemplifies how pain and sickness has undermined her energies to maintain her digital skills.) Long-term carers are also likely to face difficulties in doing things online, if they have been away from any workplace for many years.

In rural areas, people depend even more on online access both for health services and shopping. Rural Action Derbyshire is training volunteer 'digital champions', working with community organisations to offer support in village halls.[12] Generations Working Together, a Scottish organisation, develops intergenerational projects between schools and care homes or seniors' groups. An interesting case study is Roar Do Digital in Renfrewshire,[13] in which school students provided one-to-one support to seniors with tablets and laptops. Similar work has

---

[12] https://www.ruralactionderbyshire.org.uk/Blog/opening-the-door-to-the-digital-world

[13] https://generationsworkingtogether.org/case-studies/roar-do-digital

been done by the charity Generation Exchange in Haringey and Enfield.[14]

Many seniors' groups are pressing for paper and phone communications to be retained by public services and businesses. Shockingly, Council Tax reduction and Housing Benefit can only be claimed online by 31 per cent of London local authorities (Age UK, 2023). Community radio may be a useful alternative way to provide information without the cost of printing. For example, Grey Matters Productions in Brighton provides information about local seniors' services and events alongside entertainment featuring seniors' voices and reminiscences, in a fortnightly programme on a local station, RadioReverb.[15]

Health advice and peer-group messaging to reduce the need for care

Drinking less, not smoking, good diet and exercise, and keeping the brain active, are familiar recommendations for preserving good health as we age. Social connections are important for *implementing* them; people tend to do what their peers do and suggest. Exercise habits and to some extent diet are influenced by friendship networks and community facilities.

As noted by NHS England in advice to clinicians, the voluntary sector has a potential role in peer support for long-term conditions[16] and in preventive health messaging. Through participation in peer support groups, which can be phone-based, even very frail or housebound people have found opportunities to help each other, gaining self-esteem and social contacts (Boneham and Sixsmith, 2006; Gray and Worlledge, 2018). In 2013, Timebanking UK engaged several dozen GPs in 'social prescribing' of visits by timebank members to provide selected patients with emotional and practical support, and promoted many self-help groups to manage long-term conditions. Such

---

[14] Enfield Dispatch, 10 June 2021, https://enfielddispatch.co.uk/exchange-of-views/
[15] Brighton and Hove Arts Council, *Grey Matters Productions*, https://www.bh-arts.org.uk/members_all/grey-matters-productions/
[16] https://www.england.nhs.uk/long-read/peer-support/

groups could help seniors beset with common afflictions of ageing like arthritis and diabetes. A timebank covering 14 Lancashire villages (Boyle and Bird, 2014) set up self-help groups and offered alternative therapies. They also provided shopping, errands and befriending to carers referred by a carer support scheme.

Reducing poverty

Poverty is associated with health inequalities and the appearance of disability early in middle age. Average healthy life expectancy varies from 51.9 years in the most deprived tenth of small Census areas in England to 70.7 years in the least deprived tenth (Whitty, 2023).

Poverty among seniors is likely to rise in future years even if the 'triple lock' on pension updating is maintained. More seniors are still paying rent or mortgages on entering retirement, and rents are soaring (Centre for Ageing Better, 2022). Median weekly income levels of £775 for couples without children and £519 for singles compare with £561 for pensioner couples and £267 for single pensioners (Office for National Statistics, 2023b). Pensioners, like other low-income households, are disproportionately affected by the rapidly rising costs of energy and food, which take up more of their spending than for better-off households.

Help from friends and volunteers through solidarity projects can take the edge off several aspects of poverty, for example:

- helping people apply for benefits, or access appropriate advice: Pension Credit is unclaimed by an estimated 850,000 eligible pensioners;
- helping people get online: Age UK (2024b) found that around two-fifths of UK seniors cannot make fully effective use of the internet, and 1.8 million cannot use it at all. The internet gives access to cheaper utility bills, easier and higher-interest banking, easy bargain-hunting for many products, and much free entertainment. It is also increasingly important for accessing health services;
- offering lifts: even with free bus passes and subsidised taxis, seniors with mobility problems may spend a fortune on taxis;

- 'handyperson' support with minor repairs, avoiding contractors' bills and possibly worsening housing conditions if the householder cannot afford repairs in time;
- addressing fuel poverty, through information and signposting to energy-saving advice and grants, and help with DIY jobs like draught insulation and clearing a loft for contractors' insulation work.

Suitable housing for older age

As shown in Appendix B, bathing and use of stairs are among the most common physical difficulties for seniors. Home adaptations like walk-in showers, downstairs bathrooms or stair lifts could avoid some needs for homecare or for moving house.

These are examples of how age-friendly design of housing could reduce the extent of unmet need. Sadly, the UK government has allowed inflation to erode the Disability Facilities Grant which helps with home adaptations, by as much as 30 per cent since 2018.[17] But many seniors could borrow against the value of their home through equity release schemes. The obstacle may be adequate advice to do this wisely, and the problem of project management of major building works like a bathroom refit. Much has been written about 'assistive technology' for seniors, but little about the issues they face about managing house repairs and alterations if no relative is available to support them. One provision of the Care Act 2014 permits local authorities to make a loan, payable on the borrower's death, for residential care fees. However, there is no such provision for works to the home which might avoid entry into residential care. A paradox of the housing market is that while 60 per cent of seniors are home-owners, very often of a two-storey house with a garden, many families with children live in flats on upper floors without access to a private garden. Voluntary swaps, perhaps even across tenures, would help to address this issue. But local authorities and housing providers would need to set up systems to facilitate it.

---

[17] The Canary (online blog), 9 February 2024, https://www.thecanary.co/uk/2024/02/09/benefits-grants-disabled-people/

Housing aspects of the 'age-friendly communities' agenda are especially important for reducing the need for care services. Greater Manchester has sought to develop a good offer of age-friendly housing, in four ways (Greater Manchester Combined Authority, 2021): improving the quality of existing sheltered housing in terms of space and amenities; more extra-care housing, by trebling the number of extra-care flats since 2014, mostly at 'affordable' rents; ensuring accessibility standards in many new-build developments; and a big drive to offer home adaptations. Helping people stay in their existing homes as far as possible is seen as a way of reducing the need for residential care or specialist housing. Manchester is researching seniors' housing needs, investigating the scale and type of adaptations and repairs needed in existing homes.

'Extra-care' housing, with care services 'on tap' for individuals who need them, is slightly cheaper than residential care, providing a much better quality of life if it is well designed and managed (Croucher et al, 2006; Darton et al, 2008). Sheltered housing for seniors is an environment which can generate considerable mutual aid between neighbours; some examples are offered in Appendix C. It needs a community of mixed levels of dependency, and organised social activities to bring people together (Gray, 2015).

However, land for seniors' housing developments is expensive in large cities like London, limiting expansion of such provision in areas close to where many people need it. A possible innovation would be a 'network supported housing scheme'. Seniors living in the same area of a few streets could be supported to stay in their existing homes, which many would prefer, coming together for commissioning care services, cleaning and home maintenance, and socialising. They could have a support worker to help organise this, and to lean on for advice and emergencies. Some housing associations already offer a regular 'check-up' visit from a support worker to people living in ordinary community housing. Something like the care cooperative and micro-enterprise models described in Chapter 4 could facilitate this, using personal care budgets.

Another promising housing solution, though so far on a tiny scale, is 'shared lives' in which someone needing support becomes a lodger, looked after in another household. This cannot provide nursing or personal care, but may be a good solution for those with learning disabilities, sensory impairment or early-stage memory loss. 'Shared lives' is used by over 12,000 people in the UK, around one in ten being seniors.[18]

Housing and healthcare services perhaps need to be better linked up. Savings to health and social care costs could be 7.5 times the amount invested in home adaptations and services to prevent falls by seniors and disabled people (Public Health Wales, 2019). Demos (2023) estimated that investment in better domestic heating and home insulation would save up to four times as much in health treatment costs. Community projects can contribute to both falls prevention and warmer homes, as mentioned earlier. Fuel poverty is especially an issue in rural areas of northern Britain, receiving special attention for example in North Yorkshire, where community groups are recognised by the council as important channels of information.[19] Derbyshire used its public health budget in 2013–16 to improve access to affordable warmth, including advice, insulation and boiler replacement (Derbyshire County Council, 2013). In Cornwall, energy advice and 'warm homes' grants have prevented many hospital admissions.[20]

Better quality care means less care to fund?

Outcome-based commissioning often leads to reduction of the hours of formal homecare needed, as mentioned in Chapter 4. Switching attention to quality of life rather than simply addressing difficulties with ADLs, it offers support in flexible ways, tailored to clients' goals. Its emphasis is on rehabilitation and maximising independence, building on clients' 'strengths' in terms of family

---

[18] NHS (undated), https://www.nhs.uk/conditions/social-care-and-support-guide/care-services-equipment-and-care-homes/shared-lives-schemes/; and Social Care Institute for Excellence information page, https://www.scie.org.uk/housing/role-of-housing/promising-practice/models/shared-lives/

[19] North Yorkshire Council, https://www.northyorks.gov.uk/housing-and-homelessness/other-housing-information/energy-efficiency-advice/energy-efficiency-advice-ryedale/tackling-fuel-poverty-ryedale-area

[20] Cornwall County Council, https://inclusioncornwall.co.uk/winter-wellbeing/ and https://www.cornwall.gov.uk/health-and-social-care/public-health/public-health-campaigns/winter-wellbeing/

and community resources that can support them. It lends itself to the 'care team' approach advocated by Limbrick (2016) and practised by the Equal Care Coop, mentioned in Chapter 4.

Outcomes-based commissioning is closely linked to preventive approaches which draw on community projects. An example is the Neighbourhood Cares Pilot, run in two districts in Cambridgeshire in 2017–19 (Cambridgeshire County Council, 2019). Loosely based on the Buurtzorg model from the Netherlands, it involved teams of social workers and other professionals tailoring support to the clients' expressed needs, looking to see if preventive measures would prevent their needs from increasing. Some clients were seniors, others younger people with physical disabilities. The team's approach covered benefits advice and home adaptations and introduced clients to community projects that might help them. Several issues were addressed outside the usual scope of 'care', such as helping clients negotiate with a housing provider, organising repairs of domestic equipment or moving furniture. Some clients avoided admission to hospital or residential care, and built links with volunteer projects that reduced their need for formal services, especially by helping family carers to socialise more and raise their morale. Many carers were enabled to have respite breaks or stay in paid work. Neighbourhood Care held open access sessions in a public library and a doctor's surgery, and promoted volunteering. New community projects were set up, for example, a diabetic peer support group, a 'tuk-tuk' service for people who could not use standard public transport, and the Soham Community Association. The latter organised lunch meetings for community groups to come together and discuss needs and future projects. Learnings from the pilot led the council to adopt a local 'place-based' approach to commissioning social care services, drawing together public and voluntary sector services and using libraries as information hubs.

A note of caution about outcomes-based commissioning is that although this approach has been described as 'user-centred' or 'community-centred' in policy guidance from 2006–7, if budgets are stretched there is a risk that this could become distorted (Bovaird and Willis, 2012). For example, the local authority or care provider may want the client to achieve greater independence, thus needing fewer services, while the client prioritises choice and control. Manchester, in adopting a similar approach which is described as 'strengths-based commissioning', emphasises a commitment to co-production with residents which can help to avoid this problem (Manchester Local Care Organisation, 2023).

The role of seniors' networks: Manchester and Leeds

Manchester and Leeds offer valuable examples of how seniors' voices have been mobilised through older people's networks to co-produce age-friendly policies.

Seniors' organisations have much to contribute to good care policy design, to other 'age-friendly communities' policies, and to development and effective use of community support. Greater Manchester provides core funding for the regional Manchester Older People's Network,[21] which all individuals over 50 and relevant organisations can join. With 430 members, it has working groups to develop policy ideas in social care, housing and transport. It has produced housing and transport manifestos, and recommendations for health and social care. Many of the Network's suggestions have found their way into the policies described here.

Leeds is another 'age-friendly community'. It offers a good example of how to develop social networking through existing voluntary sector projects at lower cost than the 'Circles' or 'Cares' projects described in Chapter 5. The objectives are to reduce isolation and loneliness, improve health, wellbeing and engagement with local communities and official bodies, and provide more choice and control for seniors. Thirty-seven Neighbourhood Networks, each covering a city area or outlying village, are grafted onto a variety of existing organisations, including seniors' clubs or action groups, branches of national charities, and voluntary service centres (Bimpson et al 2023; Centre for Ageing Better, 2020, 2023; Sheffield Hallam University, 2022). Each organisation offers a different menu of social activities and volunteer-run support. Examples include tea and chat, lunch clubs, home help and handyperson services, digital skills classes, carer support,

---

[21] Greater Manchester Older People's Network, https://www.gmopn.org.uk/our-work

intergenerational projects with schools, advice and form-filling, holiday trips, lifts and shopping, support with long-term health conditions, and a home library service. Membership is free and individual networks have on average around 700 members. Launched in 2018 with five years' council core funding which works out at about £85 per member, they raise on average 61 per cent of their funds through additional grant applications and local activities. This includes fee income from project services of £52 per member (Dayson et al, 2022), plus fundraising activities like fairs, sales and raffles, which are regarded as sociable and enjoyable. Total funding from all sources was £199 per member, compared to £320 for the Rochdale Circle, including £30 membership subscription. Haringey Circle in its early years cost about the same in grant funding per member as the Leeds Networks, but had a high membership fee, later dropped because it was a barrier to expansion.

Conclusion

What would a good local care landscape look like in 2035–40?

A Neighbourhood Care model could be combined with the Leeds concept of Neighbourhood Networks, based on existing voluntary sector organisations, and developing micro-enterprise and social enterprises. These would provide a wide choice of personal assistants, the majority probably self-employed. They would be paid at the higher end of care assistant rates, reflecting the current demand in 2024 for a £15 wage. Personal assistants, day and respite services would be sought to suit a wide variety of needs and cultural backgrounds.

A social work team would match people in need of support to personal assistants and to other local services provided by volunteers or not-for-profit organisations. Their other roles would include:

- advice and advocacy, including on retirement housing options, home adaptations, benefits, access to GPs, dentists and other health services;
- preventive conversations for people worried about their future because of declining health or impending hospitalisation;

- help with setting up and managing personal budgets after care assessment;
- community development work to support the Neighbourhood Networks, facilitating their funding and recruitment of volunteers, identifying gaps in provision of services and activities and seeing how they could be filled.

The Neighbourhood Networks would offer a wide range of collective facilities for socialising, leisure, exercise groups, community gardening and digital skills support. Their base might be in community centres, halls attached to places of worship, libraries, health centres, cafes or pubs. They would include some intergenerational settings. They would provide carers' hubs for peer support and socialising, information and advice services including benefits advice and form-filling help. Clients would be able to choose face-to-face, online or telephone support. Core support funding would be provided for the Neighbourhood Networks, which would include seniors' membership organisations to promote and defend collective facilities and provide a voice for seniors in neighbourhood and housing planning. These would work with parallel organisations for disabled people.

Community development workers with the Neighbourhood Networks would foster community organisations to promote mutual aid, possibly involving an element of social enterprise. A central support service would offer Disclosure and Barring Service checks and training for volunteers whose role required it. Community centres, existing volunteer organisations, health centres or council buildings could provide a physical base with office facilities for mutual aid groups and social enterprises.

The choice of boundaries for neighbourhood networks needs some thought. Areas including a cross-section of the community by housing type and socio-economic status are most likely to produce a flow of volunteers, given the experience of mutual aid groups that activism and leadership tends to come from areas with above average income and educational status. Special attention is needed for under-served migrant communities, which need to be better connected to the mainstream and to public services. This presents a challenge to help them work together for effective services with indigenous British groups and members of the global majority who have been settled for generations.

Development of support for each person and their family carer, if they have one, would focus on the outcomes that are important for them rather than just on their ADL and instrumental activities of daily living capacities. Professional care teams would bring together family members with friends and volunteers, seeking to avoid excessive reliance on a family carer wherever possible through community support. The 'team owner' (the client) or family carer could decide whom she or he trusts, while the professional worker could keep an eye on any associated safeguarding risks.

Housing adaptations and improvements would be made easily available to help people stay in their existing homes, if they wanted to, rather than move to residential care or find a sheltered housing option that might mean moving away from friends and familiar settings. While the stock of sheltered or fully accessible housing may be limited, and fixed at least in the medium term, much can be achieved by using it flexibly. For example, seniors who own an unsuitable home could benefit from an exchange system, possibly including exchange across tenures so that they could move to social-rented sheltered accommodation and be supported to sell or rent out their existing home. A brokerage organisation to help people move, or to sell, repair, adapt or insulate their home is needed, which could arrange contractors for them and sometimes project management. It could help seniors arrange suitable credit facilities, either through equity release or through a local authority charge which would eventually be repaid from their estate.

This kind of neighbourhood plan builds on the local examples in this chapter, on the material about solidarity projects presented in Chapter 6, and on the examples of non-profit provision from Chapter 4. It could be built through co-production processes based on the Manchester example, within an overall 'age-friendly community' approach.

8

Conclusions and solutions

Introduction

The overall conclusion of this book is that expanding informal support from beyond the family is crucial to helping both family carers and seniors, especially those without close relatives to hand. Informal support must engage the wider community to keep up with rising needs. The need for better and cheaper formal services needs to be pushed forward in tandem; paid carers are needed especially for personal care. Formal and informal care are complements; there is limited substitutability between personal care from formal services or close relatives and support from non-kin. Both need to expand. Community engagement with informal care can drive forward a consciousness of the importance of better formal services and political pressure to raise their priority in national budgets.

Advocates of free tax-funded care argue that it ensures equality by health status as well as income. A gradual transition to free universal care could be achieved in stages; the suggestions of Chapter 4 are summarised in what follows. But abolishing charges would consume far less money than the vital requirements of helping more people with more hours, and paying care workers adequately. Plans for the future of formal care services need to consider that much higher care workers' pay is needed to sustain an adequate workforce, and to recognise the trade-offs between different objectives; making care more affordable, increasing hours offered per client, the number of clients reached or the needs threshold, the quality of care services, and the extent of support given to intensive family carers. Lower unit costs and better quality of care could be achieved by expanding non-profit provision and outcomes-based approaches.

Summarising the main messages of previous chapters:

- The care system is very heavily dependent on unpaid care, which involves over nine times more carers than the paid sector, and is over four times its value, according to varying estimates (Chapter 2). The state could never afford to replace it all.
- Informal (unpaid) care is falling on fewer and fewer shoulders, for demographic and labour market reasons (Chapters 2 and 3). This creates unacceptable stress. We need to involve more people in informal care. Friends, neighbours and volunteers could ease the load, but they cannot take on the core tasks of personal care, which must be a priority for state services. Seniors without available relatives have a serious lack of informal support, childlessness is growing, and the longer people live, the more likely they are to outlast their partner and their friends.
- Carers need more support (Chapter 3); cash and services from the state; support with domestic tasks, errands, social life and moral support from the community; better carer's leave from employers. Carer's Allowance should be made into a proper income for paid work (Chapter 4). Carers' needs have important social and emotional aspects; community groups and community centres can help, and provide settings for peer support (Chapter 5).
- Growing community support and informal care beyond the family needs to go much further than the tiny role of traditional volunteering, which however received an important boost during the COVID-19 pandemic. Chapter 5 presents a vision of the 'caring economy' or 'commons of care', involving development of mutual aid and other solidarity projects, and reducing social isolation. Chapter 6 continues this theme, suggesting that the history of mutual aid groups, most recently in the pandemic, shows important potential for the future. Timebanks, which have been promoted as a form of mutual aid, are rather less successful at that but have a role in enlarging

people's personal networks and supporting community projects, centres and services.
- Chapter 7 locates community solidarity within a preventive agenda. We need to stay healthy to need less care. Avoiding loneliness, keeping socially and physically active, are an important part of the battle, in which personal friendship networks and community projects have an important role. Also important is minimising barriers to daily living for disabled or age-affected people. 'Age-Friendly Communities' policies provide a useful holistic framework for a preventive approach which makes good use of community strengths and resources, a theme continued later in this chapter.

The future cost of care

Chapter 4 estimates at over £52 billion, in 2023 prices, the likely cost of offering a national care service to all those who are in substantial need according to Care Act criteria, and who would be likely to take up personal care if it was free. It includes homecare plus the 'care' element of residential places. For comparison, local authorities spent £20.5 billion net, plus user charges of over £3.2 billon (ADASS, 2024).

Obviously if charges were retained, demand would be smaller, but interpreting the estimates of the New Economics Foundation and Women's Budget Group (NEF/WBG) paper (Bedford and Button, 2022) to which Chapter 4 refers, extra demand generated by abolishing charges would only raise costs by about 4 per cent[1] over their 'baseline' scenario. Extra demand from people who are not currently local authority clients would likely be small; Scottish experience suggests only 29 per cent of seniors with substantial needs actually took up free personal homecare when it was introduced. With the £15 hourly carer's wage suggested in Chapter 4, the cost of making care free would be less than £7 billion.

Thus, it must be emphasised that most of the cost increase is not due to making care free. It is badly needed to help more people

---

[1] Based on author's interpretation of Table 5 in the technical annex to Bedford and Button (2022).

and pay staff better. NEF/WBG estimate that to provide for all those with severe needs even without the small extra demand induced by making care free would increase the number of clients by around 200,000 over-65s and 183,000 younger adults,[2] adding 39 per cent to what local authorities actually spent in 2021/2. (That was £22.11 billion, according to ADASS [2022a].) NEF/WBG also factor in an average care package for homecare of 12 hours rather than ten, and payment for care workers' travel time.

A substantial pay rise for care workers is not only fair; it is also needed to recruit to the care sector, which in March 2024 had 131,000 vacancies (Samuel, 2024). The estimates in Chapter 4 assume an average wage rate of £15 per hour. The jump from the National Living Wage of £11.44 of 2023/4 (barely reached in 2023 by many care workers) to £15 would make a difference of just over a fifth to total costs, since labour costs are around 70 per cent.

If staff are recruited from overseas or from economic inactivity, rather than from other UK jobs, the extra taxes they would pay would offset part of the cost. Further modelling is needed to estimate this factor, as well as the considerable potential savings of better care to the NHS.

How does Scotland afford free personal care, in particular extending entitlements from over-65s to all adults in 2019? Scotland in 2021 spent £474 on adult social care per head of the population, compared to £550 in Northern Ireland, £494 in Wales and only £372 in England (Dodsworth and Oung, 2023). So despite free personal care, Scotland spent less than Wales or Northern Ireland. Obviously spending per head reflects levels of need and provider costs, not just the scope or quality of service. But the difference in care spending is partly driven by political choice.

In 2019, extending the 2002 policy of free personal care for seniors to all adults in Scotland required planning to raise the care budget by a further one-fifth (Feeley, 2021). This was the choice that Scotland accepted. Feeley estimated that a further

---

[2] Client figures for 2022/3 taken from King's Fund blog, https://www.kingsfund.org.uk/insight-and-analysis/long-reads/social-care-360-access#2.-receipt-of-social-care; comparison from Bedford and Button (2022).

£100 million would be needed for each £1 added to carers' hourly wage, which by 2022/3 was a minimum of only £12 per hour.[3]

Planning the budget is far from simple. Although Scottish social care expenditure around doubled between 2004 and 2018 (Independent Age, 2020), local authorities reduced some other services to fund the new right to free personal care for over-65s, and long waiting lists developed, as explained in Chapter 3. A further difficulty which has arisen in planning the Scottish National Care Service is the high and somewhat unpredictable cost of 'levelling up' standards and practices across many different local authorities. Fears of escalating costs due to this concern have held up the establishment of a unified national care service, now not expected until 2027–9.[4]

Pathways towards greater funding and lower charging

Appendix A suggests several ways of raising extra public money to pay for social care in England, mainly through taxing wealth and reducing tax concessions to wealthier individuals. But only a share of extra revenue can be used for social care; the currently emasculated state of public services means that there will be many competing demands on additional revenue sources. Expansion of formal care on the scale suggested in Chapter 4 is a crucial priority, but it will take some time, not least because of staff shortages as well as funding.

Chapter 4 suggests two measures as possible stepping stones towards universal free care, both for homecare and in residential settings:

- A weekly cap on the number of hours of care that someone pays for. For anyone whose needs exceeded the cap, extra hours would be free. This resembles the Welsh £120 weekly cap described in Chapter 4, but it needs to be inflation-proofed

---

[3] https://www.gov.scot/publications/adult-social-care-workers-minimum-pay/
[4] BBC Scotland, 14 December 2023, https://www.bbc.co.uk/news/uk-scotland-67714086; and BBC News, 12 July 2023, https://www.bbc.co.uk/news/uk-scotland-scotland-politics-66176124

by index-linking, perhaps to the Real Living Wage (the level defined by the Living Wage Foundation[5]), so that its value in hours would be maintained. The cap could be reduced gradually over time, increasing the free element.
- Increasing the state-funded element of personal budgets by enough to pay for extra hours for people who rely heavily on an unpaid carer. They could use this either to pay the unpaid carer (if permitted by a change in regulations), or someone else, as the family chooses.

The free element of care packages could be gradually increased over time. Its feasible size depends not only on overall national budget constraints but on choices about how much to spend on quality improvements, investment in workforce training and new provider capacity, preventive health measures and, perhaps most importantly, care workers' pay level. This raises the question of equity between low-paid care workers and the wealthier service users. Some users have no savings, after being unable to work for years, or, increasingly, still pay market rents during retirement. But others have ample savings after well-paid careers.

Some variation of the free care ration according to users' financial status would be possible. However the minimum savings level at which co-payments begin, defined as £23,250 ever since 2010, badly needs updating. But inequalities can best be addressed through taxes on *all wealthier people*, rather than what is, in effect, a tax just on the sick or disabled.

Support for informal carers

To reward and encourage informal carers, co-resident household members could be allowed to receive, as a wage, the personal budget of the person they support. Under current regulations, household members cannot generally be hired as personal assistants. A family member who is juggling part-time care with part-time work might find it attractive to take on say 12 hours' weekly care work at the rate an agency-sourced personal assistant would charge.

---

[5] Living Wage Foundation, https://livingwage.org.uk/what-real-living-wage

Conclusions and solutions

Chapter 4 suggests a sum of £16.2 billion (gross) to support intensive family carers by transforming Carer's Allowance into a payment for work, at least for part of their hours. This could be in addition to letting them use their relative's personal budget if both people prefer that to having formal homecare. The *net cost*, if both Carer's Allowance and Attendance Allowance were absorbed into a new payment, would be just £5.7 million. Paying carers for what they do would not only be fair but would probably save public funds; family carers do not need agency overheads. Local pilots might help to see whether this would also reduce demand for residential care, which absorbs 57.5 per cent of English local authorities' gross care budgets (King's Fund, 2024b).

Intensive carers also need a right to periods of time off; a right to respite care, and longer carer's leave, preferably paid, from employers. The UK's five days, unpaid, is well behind some other countries, as noted in Chapter 3. It seems unjust that paid maternity leave is available for 39 weeks, but carer's leave is often unpaid and so short.

Carers' voices, heard in a community project described in Chapter 5, expressed a demand for more information, facilities and spaces for peer support, respite care, opportunities for peer support and socialising, advice and advocacy on benefits and housing issues. One might add day centre services, training and counselling. Informal care by close relatives could be more easily sustained if these needs were better met.

Supply-side measures to reduce the cost of formal care

Chapter 4 describes possible ways of reducing non-wage costs of formal care while improving quality of outcomes for service users:

- Micro-enterprises, care cooperatives and social enterprises could reduce unit costs compared to corporate agencies, by reducing overheads and removing shareholder profits. There is evidence that they often offer a better-quality service, while permitting higher care workers' pay at given costs per client.
- Cost savings in homecare, and greater client satisfaction, can be achieved by 'outcome-based commissioning' of care; giving care workers more autonomy to provide what clients want

rather than doing a pre-arranged, fixed set of tasks. Pilots of this system, as described in Chapters 4 and 7, have often discovered that clients need less support than had been expected. Hospital or residential care admissions are reduced. Advocates of outcomes-based commissioning often stress the advantages of *early* help; its medical aspects are appropriate diet and exercise, effective management of long-term health conditions, while its social aspects are finding activities that offer pleasure and a sense of purpose, within a supportive friendship circle.

- Use of expensive residential care needs to be minimised, by helping people stay in their own homes if possible, which is what most of them prefer. Home adaptations, and/or local networks of care-needers sharing some support services can support this objective. Where more support is needed, extra-care housing, mentioned in Chapters 4 and 7, is likely to be cheaper and more congenial than a residential care home.

The nature of care as a relationship

Social care can be conceptualised both quantitatively and qualitatively. This text has attempted to balance the two approaches. While the quantitative perspective is important to define the scale of the care deficit, both formal and informal, there is also a qualitative dimension, highlighted in Chapter 5, which must be addressed by thinking of care as a set of relationships. These relationships have an emotional dimension, implying a need for friendship and the avoidance of loneliness. Increasingly, support to participate in social life is being recognised as very important, which is where community solidarity comes in.

Community informants mentioned in Chapter 5 wanted formal care provision to allow for development of relationships between carer and service user, requiring continuity, flexibility and sufficient time for social interaction, attending to emotional needs. Echoing Kartupelis' concept of 'relational care', their wishes stand in stark contrast to the 15-minute or 30-minute visits by constantly changing agency staff which characterise much formal homecare delivered by current corporate agencies, operating with the very low prices per hour that local authorities can currently afford. 'Relational care' is better reflected in the approach of micro-enterprise and non-profit organisations described in Chapter 4. They can improve the quality of care by developing understanding and responsive relationships with clients and flexibility according to their needs. They can work together with community projects based on mutual aid principles and co-production.

How community solidarity can help

Formal care for seniors is largely concerned with 'personal care', which friends or neighbours do not do. Particularly with the current rationing of a stretched budget, seniors' care packages focus mainly on bedroom and bathroom tasks, although the option of personal budgets offers some flexibility about what is covered. Scottish care statistics show that personal care is over 90 per cent of homecare in Scotland. However, the remaining tenth consists of things like meal preparation, shopping and day-time respite care, tasks which unpaid non-family helpers can support. Several other important needs are simply not covered by formal care: home maintenance, gardening, befriending, accompanying and lifts. Digital skills support has barely entered the scope of formal care services except where health boards have addressed its role in accessing health services, but it is a most important offering of friends, younger relatives and community projects.

The contribution of non-kin is more for support with instrumental activities of daily living rather than activities of daily living; the range of unmet needs which make the difference between short-term survival and quality of life. Non-relatives can support family carers, isolated singles and formal services in many important ways, especially at the stage in later life trajectories where *prevention* and sustaining quality of life can help to arrest further age-related decline.

Community solidarity belongs to an agenda of early help and prevention, helping to fill gaps in formal support. While basic physical functioning for seniors depends on formal services, especially for those who live alone, quality of life depends on informal support which is crucial to social inclusion and to avoiding the vicious circle of inactivity, loneliness, lack of purpose and worsening health. Thus, models of care as a relationship, within a 'caring society' or 'caring economy', need to inform an agenda for 'ageing well' with minimal care. Care as friendship, rather than as unpaid 'tasks', may be best achieved in informal settings rather than contractual volunteering.

Widening the caring circle: the importance of friendship networks

Chapter 3 emphasises the importance of non-family support for people with neither partners nor grown-up children, although inevitably they are more dependent on formal services. Chapter 5 shows how good instrumental support requires a large and varied friendship network, including people with different skill sets and contacts. The people most likely to lack friend and neighbour support are newcomers to an area, lone parents and intensive carers. Seniors need some younger friends; their peer group naturally fades away as age advances.

Also important to friendship formation are absence of crime, housing and street designs that lend themselves to neighbour contact, and having plenty of congenial meeting places like community centres, cafes, pubs, sociable parks and shopping places. These aspects of an inclusive, friendly social and physical environment are supported by some of the 'age-friendly communities' policies described in Chapter 7.

Looking at projects to help isolated people expand their networks and generate mutual aid, Chapter 5 notes that the achievements of the Cares Family of projects, and most of the Circles set up by Hilary Cottam, have come at very high cost in grant aid. Chapter 7 presents the Leeds Neighbourhood Networks as a less costly and highly effective alternative model.

How community solidarity can contribute to a prevention and early help agenda

Turning from friendship networks to community projects as a source of extra-familial support, Chapter 6 focuses on the achievements and future potential of four types of organisations which can contribute to the development of the 'caring economy' or 'commons of care'.

Conclusions and solutions

Mutual aid groups like those of the pandemic period, if revived, could have an important role in supporting 'early help and prevention' policies through several kinds of help which are important ancillaries to formal services. This would not, however, attempt to replace the essential core of 'personal care' from formal services, which needs to be preserved and expanded. Help to individuals with some non-personal care needs could be arranged by links between their professional personal assistant, doctor or social worker and a community project, taking up the idea of a 'care team' (Limbrick, 2016) which brings together formal care, family, friends and volunteers. This concept is also used by the Equal Care coop (mentioned in Chapter 4), with the emphasis on the client as 'team owner'.

Projects based on mutual aid principles can also support many kinds of collective facilities: community centres, carers' hubs, day services and lunch clubs, social activities in sheltered housing schemes, digital skills learning, health prevention and peer support groups, translation and community transport. They could work in conjunction with non-profit providers, whether micro-enterprises, care cooperatives or social enterprises. The care sector contains about 5,000 social enterprises across England. Many achieve high quality provision, over half of them in running day services and many engaging volunteers (Hall, 2022; Hall and Alexander, 2023). As described in Chapter 6, timebanks' role in bringing people together and running community centres, community gardens, lunch clubs and other group activities has been rather more successful than their role in person-to-person support, which has high staff costs due to the need for safeguarding, people-matching and supervision.

The mutual aid movement and timebanking share some key principles of reciprocity and co-production, flexibility of response to the needs of those supported, and equality of status between helpers and helped. Reciprocity in this context means that everyone tries to contribute whatever they can, whether in time and services, or goods and money. These principles are an important legacy which gives dignity and self-esteem to all parties, allowing them to express their needs. They avoid the excessive formalism and boundaries of particular roles which characterises some traditional volunteering. For example, the 'befriender' in some schemes for volunteers to visit housebound seniors is instructed not to stray into other activities like shopping, even if the client wants them; but this is hardly in the flexible spirit of 'outcome-based commissioning' which has been applauded in relation to formal services.

The NHS Responder scheme, as a contrasting example of traditional 'top-down' volunteering, illustrates some limitations of the traditional approach, but with several hundred thousand people involved, also a huge uptick in mobilising community effort which may be positively developed in coming years. Recent reports mentioned in Chapter 6 suggest that it is moving in a more flexible direction to respond to a greater variety of user-led requests.

The fourth organisational type, the community union ACORN, shows impressive examples of solidarity outside of workplace issues with users of many kinds of service. It works by researching needs, lobbying and occasionally engaging in street protests to support people in dispute with landlords or council services. It exemplifies an important political role of groups based on mutual aid principles.

An expansion of mutual aid might be stimulated by community centres, residents' associations, seniors' organisations or faith groups. Younger volunteers need to be brought in as well as retired people. Possible recruitment channels include councils for voluntary service, national charities, student groups and religious congregations. The Leeds Neighbourhood Networks mentioned in Chapter 7 are an example of how an array of seniors' groups based on existing voluntary sector organisations can be brought together to provide a city-wide resource for social activities, information and advice, and some mutual aid services. Together with promotion of effective intergenerational mutual aid projects, this would help to realise Peter Limbrick's vision of 'care activism' (Limbrick, 2016). Limbrick has been criticised for over-optimism about the availability of volunteers (Sutherland, 2017). The challenges of engaging large numbers of people in solidaristic action should not be under-estimated. But the experiences of COVID-19 pandemic-period mutual aid, and the continued activity of around 200,000 volunteers who supported the NHS Volunteer Responder scheme, offer counterweight to Sutherland's pessimism. As shown in Chapter 5, the volunteer requirements of a typical urban street appear actually quite small.

Reducing the demand for care services: preventive health measures, solidarity and an age-friendly environment

Reducing the demand for care may appear to be passing responsibility from public services to the individual. Indeed, if we all took perfect care of ourselves as we age, we would be less likely to become dependent. But poverty, poor housing and fuel poverty, lack of support from absent or non-existent relatives, ageism, poor public transport and difficulty in accessing an ever more digitalised and stretched health service stand in the way of this for many. All these aspects of public policy need to be addressed to keep demand for care in check.

The 'age-friendly communities' movement is a useful framework for holistic development of policies which support ageing with minimal difficulty, offering some local examples of good practice described in Chapter 7. The eight domains of the 'age-friendly communities' framework can all contribute to reducing care demand and there are opportunities for community solidarity projects to support each of them, shown in Table 8.1.

The domain of social inclusion is an important and overarching one. To be of genuine benefit to those affected, improving their quality of life, policy developments need to be grounded in a co-production framework which gives them voice and agency. At the 'micro' level of the individual care-needer, outcomes-focused commissioning and a strengths-based approach offers scope for reducing demand for formal care through making best use of community resources, including the kind of solidarity projects described in Chapter 6. Recommendations about how these various elements could be brought together have been offered in Chapter 7 through an imagined vision of a 'caring neighbourhood', reflecting the ideas of the Care Collective (Chapter 5), and the suggestions for non-profit care provision (Chapter 4).

Table 8.1: The eight policy domains of 'age-friendly communities'[1] and how community projects can contribute

Domain	Community projects' potential contribution
1. Outdoor spaces and buildings	Shaping policies for accessible and age/disability-friendly parks, streets, shopping malls and public buildings, through walkabouts, surveys, consultations and conversations with service managers. Organised walks or exercise in parks. Community gardening, often in an intergenerational setting. Volunteering for park maintenance.
2. Transport	Shaping policies for bus services and stops, and for age-friendly train stations, including maintaining station staffing and ticket offices.
3. Housing	Developing mutual aid, 'good neighbour' and befriending schemes through tenants' and residents' groups. Helping to run common room activities in sheltered housing.
4. Social participation	Helping to run community activities that bring people together: community centres, lunch clubs, choirs, art groups, exercise and dance sessions, community minibus transport. Support to social enterprises that provide day-care services. Befriending services, escorting people to community events. Visiting housebound people and helping with home library services.
5. Respect and social inclusion	Seniors' groups to promote policy improvements for their age group and engage in individual advocacy; providing a voice and focus for dialogue with service providers and businesses. Intergenerational projects to bring youth and seniors together for socialising and skill sharing, transmission of historical memory and local history. Helping people access the internet for social purposes, such as Facebook, Zoom and WhatsApp.
6. Civic participation and employment	Working with trade unions to secure better carer's leave and better flexible working policies for older employees. Supporting people to sign up for a postal vote.
7. Communication and information	Provision of information on local services, benefits, social events and activities, consultations, preventive health messaging. Signposting to professional advice where needed on subjects like wills, powers of attorney, seniors' housing and care options. Helping people use online services and information sources.
8. Health services and community support	Addressing isolation and loneliness as an aid to remaining in good health and morale. Preventive health messaging. Helping people access the internet for health service communications. Ancillary support to formal care services through helping with home maintenance, shopping, cooking, lifts and helping people go out and about. Lunch clubs for sociability and healthy food.

[1] Source: Centre for Ageing Better (nd)

Community and state together building a caring economy

The demand for a free universal care service has been associated with a vision of the 'caring economy' or the 'commons of care' in which non-intimate aspects of care can become a collective community responsibility (Chatzidikis et al, 2020). Just as the mutual aid movement internationally has been a vehicle for exposing gaps in state service and pressing for more, it has a potentially important advocacy and lobbying role in relation to social care. The future development of mutual aid, and the revival of the achievements of the COVID-19 pandemic period, may depend on public awareness about care issues, but also drive it forward in an upward spiral. Greater awareness would lead to better community and individual planning for care-prevention, self-care, and care of others in our ageing society. It would recognise the need for community action alongside pressure for greater public investment and acceptance of its cost − cost not only of a care service but of community infrastructure in terms of more, and more accessible, community meeting spaces, accessible transport and housing. The ageing society needs community sharing of care and support, building a culture of caring in which responsibility for those who can't or can't any longer reciprocate is shared beyond the family. As the Manchester care strategy says, we need to prevent, reduce and delay, until later in the onset of ageing, the need for formal care. The more community action can help to do this, the better and more affordable a national care service can be. Quality adult care for all who need it is a crucial goal, for which the struggle may take some time. Alongside that struggle, we need to sustain and spread informal care, and support those who provide it; and also ensure that future pensioners will enter retirement still in good health.

APPENDIX A

Cost calculations and revenue sources for expanding subsidised care

This appendix presents an illustrative selection of measures to increase overall UK tax revenue. Some which are often advocated to fund particular programmes are omitted, like taxes on fossil fuel companies (often linked to environmental measures) or reduction of overall company tax concessions to fund better benefits. The total yield from them all would be around £60 billion to £80 billion, about 5.6 per cent to 7.5 per cent of total government spending. This compares to the budget for the NHS in 2022/3 (£212 billion), for education (£106 billion), social protection, which includes care, pensions and other cash benefits (£319 billion), defence (£56 billion), transport and 'public order and safety' (£44 billion each), housing (£18 billion) and environmental protection (£14 billion). It is being argued that the NHS needs an extra £40 billion, investments in renewable energy and home insulation around £28 billion, restoring central government grants to local government to the real-terms level of 2009/10 about £18.5 billion, restoration of the real value of cash benefits to households to its level of 2012, £21.2 billion (Rowlands, 2023), plus possibly additional sums for tax cuts on lower incomes.

Increasing revenue is not the only possibility. Many are the arguments about how large government borrowing should be allowed to grow, or which public expenditures should be cut. Subsidies to fossil fuel companies are frequently opposed by environmental campaigners; others question the need for nuclear weapon upgrades or advocate rent control as an alternative to much of the spending on housing benefits, to mention just some examples.

Appendix A

Table A1: Possible sources of tax revenue to expand social care spending

Measure	Likely annual yield	Source and comments
The Trades Union Congress proposes a once-off levy on fortunes over £3 million; rates varying from 1.7% to 3.5% for those with over £10 million	£10.4 billion	Highly prone to evasion through moving money overseas or into trusts. The Trades Union Congress' proposal was reported in the *Guardian*; calculations relate to 2023, produced by Landman Economics (Neate, 2023). Prem Sikka (2023) estimates a larger yield of £22 billion from a wealth tax of 2% on assets over £10 million, which would apply to 22,000 people
Make National Insurance payable at a standard rate on all income above the lower exemption threshold	At least £12.5 billion (Murphy, 2024), possibly up to £16.6 billion*	Currently a reduced rate of 2% is paid on income over £50,270
Tax capital gains as if they were earned income	Approximately £15 billion (Intergenerational Foundation, 2023) to £17 billion (Sikka, 2023)	Currently capital gains are taxed at 20% even if the marginal income tax rate of the taxpayer is higher. There is also an additional tax-free allowance for capital gains on top of the personal tax-free allowance for income tax
Loss of corporation tax revenue due to company strategies for shifting profits overseas	Approx £22.74 billion, of which at least £2 billion may be retrievable by government	Very frequently done by multinationals. Hard to estimate, but the average across all OECD countries may be around 1% of GDP (Cobham and Janský, 2020). Also very hard to prevent. New OECD rules from January 2024, which attempt to ensure companies pay at least 15% tax on their profits in *some* country, with a reporting basis to permit additional tax to be levied in countries where the rate is higher, are expected to increase UK tax revenue by at least £2 billion (HMRC, 2023; Nair, 2023)
Limit all tax reliefs to 20% even if the taxpayer's own marginal tax rate is higher	£14.5 billion (Sikka, 2023)	

(continued)

Table A1: Possible sources of tax revenue to expand social care spending (continued)

Measure	Likely annual yield	Source and comments
Abolish separate tax-free allowance for dividend income	£1.3 billion (Palmer et al, 2019)	Currently the allowance is £2,000
Charge National Insurance on earnings of people over state pension age who are in employment	£1.1 billion (Adam and Waters, 2018)	Currently no National Insurance is payable by people over state pension age, even if they are still working
Charge National Insurance on unearned income	£8.5 billion (Advani et al, 2021)	Currently income from interest, rent and dividends is exempt
Removing the exemption from capital gains tax on death	£1.2 billion (Corlett, 2018)	Currently no capital gains tax is payable by heirs if the deceased's chargeable assets rise in value between the date of death and the date they are distributed to heirs
Doubling council tax on the four top tax bands	£8.5 billion (Intergenerational Foundation, 2023)	Would induce downsizing by seniors living alone, and incentivise sub-letting and flat conversions

Note: * Advani et al (2021) adjusted for reduction of National Insurance contribution rate from 12% to 10% in March 2024 budget.

Table A2: Cost calculation for homecare

		All adults	Over 65	18–64
A	No. of clients with LA need[1]	2,292,000	1,642,000	650,000
B	No. of clients that one worker can serve[1]		2	1.2
C	Care workers for total homecare need[2]	1,362,667	821,000	541,667
D	Billing rate per hour[3]	£34.69		
E	Billed hours per week per worker[1]	24.2		
F	Weeks per year	52		
G	Total cost of homecare if 100 per cent of those in LA need use it	£59,485,708,949		

Appendix A

Table A2: Cost calculation for homecare (continued)

		All adults	Over 65	18–64
K	Likely take-up rate of hours if no user charges or staff shortage[4]	54.4%	49%	68%
L	Total cost if no user charges paid	£32,353,270,097		

Notes: [1] Based on Bedford and Button (2022); [2] Derived from first two rows; [3] Based on rate proposed by UK Home Care Association as necessary for viability of providers (UKHCA, 2023). Includes wage, holiday and sick pay, office costs, management staff and profit. Permits hourly wage rate of approximately £15; [4] Take-up rate in hours estimated by Bedford and Button (2022). The rate in hours is higher than the percentage of care-needers who take up a state service, as explained in Chapter 4.

Table A3: Estimated cost of residential and nursing care

A	Net expenditure on residential and nursing care in 2022/3[1]	£3,987,088,000
B	Number of clients supported in residential settings, 2022/3	372,035
C	Assumed number of hours of care in residential settings per client per week[2]	31
D	Hourly wage rate 2024[3]	£15.00
E	Labour cost per hour[4]	£17.70
F	Labour cost of care if wage at £15 per hour, for all clients[5]	£10,615,051,434
G	Overheads and profit on care element of residential service[6]	£4,776,773,145
H	Total cost of care element including overheads and profit	£15,391,824,579

Notes: [1] This row is for comparison only: a large proportion of gross expenditure is paid by clients, so this row does not indicate cost of provision. Of the total, nursing care is almost £1.4 billion and residential care £2.6 billion. [2] As assumed by Bedford and Button (2022). [3] £15 is the wage rate assumed necessary, explained in Chapter 4. [4] Add to wage National Insurance at 14% (average rate in 2022/3) plus pension 4%. [5] row B × row C × row E × 52. [6] Assume 45% of staff costs, following Bedford and Button (2022).

APPENDIX B

Seniors' different needs for help and how they are met

Table B1 shows how many seniors in each age band had difficulty with various tasks, and what proportion received some help with them. The first four columns are based on the English Longitudinal Study of Ageing (ELSA) data for 2018–19 (Banks et al, 2024), the others from the HSE (NatCen Social Research, 2023). ELSA asks if someone had a difficulty and then whether anyone helped with that task. But it does not indicate how serious the need for help was. So column E of Table B1 draws on the HSE, which does ask whether someone can do a task by themselves with difficulty, or only with help, or not at all, although its sample is much smaller. From the HSE, one can see what proportion of those with a difficulty couldn't manage without help and how many actually had help. The difference is the proportion with unmet need.

Column D shows that two of the biggest needs are help with bathing and with stairs. They are ones that might be addressed at least partly by home adaptations or housing design. The other major needs (help with going out, shopping and housework) are things that formal care services rarely provide. Extending also to gardening, these are the biggest *unmet* needs (column E) and are suitable for friends, neighbours and volunteers to take on.

ELSA data analysed by the author for Wave 9 (2018–19; Banks et al, 2024) also offer a breakdown of the types of informal helper who support the different tasks. Results for the most common types of difficulty are shown in Table B2. For each activity of daily living (ADL) or instrumental activity of daily living (IADL) with which there is difficulty, the respondent is asked whether s/he had help and from whom, distinguishing partner, son, friend, and so on. The table shows that the contribution of non-relatives, and also of grandchildren, is largely for IADLs – shopping, getting out,

Appendix B

Table B1: Help received and need for help, by age band

	Age 65–74	Age 75–84	Age 85 +	All age groups over 65	
	% who have difficulty	% who have difficulty	% who have difficulty	% who have difficulty	Unmet need with this task, % of all over 65s estimated from HSE
	A	B	C	D	E
Any task	21.2	36.8	57.5	31.0	14.1
Dressing	10.9	16.8	28.1	15.0	7.1
Bath or shower	6.8	11.4	26.9	10.7	6.1
Getting in/out of bed	5.2	7.6	13.3	7.0	5.7
Using toilet	3.3	5.4	11.8	5.0	2.3
Eating, cutting up food	1.9	3.3	8.4	3.1	2.4
Using stairs	10.9	16.8	28.1	15.0	18.1
Walking out of doors	9.7	18.5	35.1	15.8	16.2
Taking medication	1.9	4.4	15.4	4.3	1.3
Shopping for food	6.4	11.8	30.8	11.0	20.7
Housework/gardening	11.9	21.2	43.2	18.8	15.4
Managing bills, paperwork	1.7	5.9	20.1	5.3	10.6
N for this age group	3,080	1,777	443	5,300	2,254
No. who were asked about help because they had some difficulty	1,624	1,216	336	3,176	665

Source: Author's analysis of ELSA Wave 9 (2018–19) and Health Survey of England data for 2018, available through NatCen Social Research (2023)

housework and gardening, while bathroom tasks fall to partners, daughters and sons.

Table B2 shows the HSE data (NatCen Social Research, 2023) on who provided help and how this changed over the pre-COVID-19 pandemic period. Help from friends or relatives fell slightly – from almost 38 per cent of all instances of help in 2011 to 31.5 per cent in 2018. Non-relatives were 12.7 per cent of unpaid helpers of the over-65s in 2011 and 12.9 per cent in 2018 – a considerably higher proportion than the 7 per cent shown in the Family Resources Survey for helpers of people across *all ages*. For younger adults, unpaid helpers are most frequently their parents; but parent helpers are obviously rare for the over-65s.

In both years, partners of seniors were the largest category of helpers, with daughters just behind and sons the third largest, showing the significant disadvantage of being single or childless. Each category of informal help fell very slightly over the period.

The relative proportions of different informal helpers changed little from 2011 to 2018. Slightly fewer people were helped by daughters and slightly more by sons; but this relative gender shift is not statistically significant.

The proportion of the sample receiving unpaid help fell by almost 10 percentage points over 2011–18, while the proportion who needed help with any task fell by only 6.4 per cent. Yet there was no corresponding increase in receipt of formal homecare, most of which was paid for privately in both years. Many people had multiple types of help, informal and formal.

Partners who helped provided on average over 20 hours of care per week, compared to 9–13 hours from sons and daughters, 8–9 hours from other relatives, and only five hours from non-relatives. ELSA does not tell us how much of carers' time is spent doing each type of task; to investigate that reliably would need a far higher sample size.

Appendix B

Table B2: Who helps with which tasks?

Task	Percent of over-65s needing help who received it from different types of helper*						Total of people needing and receiving help with ADL/IADL
	Spouse/ partner*	Daughter	Son	Grandchild	Other relative	Friend	Neighbour	
Any task(s)	23.4	21.6	14.5	7.2	2.9	9.5	3	1,330
Washing/dressing	26.9	13.4	3.9	4.5	1.8	2.6	1	382
Eating	32.7	14.2	10	4.2	3.3	3.3	0.8	120
Mobility	18.9	22.8	11.5	6.7	3.4	7.1	2.4	496
Shopping/housework or gardening	27.4	23.3	15.1	6.9	2.5	9.3	3.1	870
Managing money	54.1	24.1	12.9	2.2	2.2	2.6	0	232
Taking medication	47.4	15.1	9.2	4.3	1.1	1.1	0.5	185

Notes: * Percentage of instances of help, corrected in the case of partners for the percentage of people with difficulty in relation to the particular task who said they could not do it without help. Some people receive help from more than one person.

Source: Author's analysis of ELSA Wave 9 (2018–19); UK Data Service (2020) *English Longitudinal Study of Ageing (ELSA) Wave 9*; see Banks et al (2024)

Table B3: Trend in contributions of different informal helpers, 2011–2018

	2011				2018			
Type of helper Total over-65s	Number recorded	Number recorded as % of over-65s	% of unpaid helpers	% of those needing help	Number recorded	Number recorded as % of over-65s	% of unpaid helpers	% of those needing help
in sample	2,075				2,254			
Partner	218	10.5	30.0	27.7	173	7.7	30.6	24.4
Son	114	5.5	15.7	14.5	98	4.3	17.3	13.8
Daughter	215	10.4	29.6	27.3	155	6.9	27.4	21.8
Other relative	87	4.2	12.0	11.1	66	2.9	11.7	9.3
Friend	60	2.9	8.3	7.6	47	2.1	8.3	6.6
Neighbour	32	1.5	4.4	4.1	26	1.2	4.6	3.7
Total informal helpers	726	35.0	100.0		565	25.1	100.0	
Total over-65s needing help	787				710			
% of sample needing help		37.9				31.5		
% of those needing help who got informal support				63.9				54.1
Have home-carer	66	3.2		8.4	65	2.9		9.2
Have cleaner	51	2.5		6.5	48	2.1		6.8
Council homecare				2.2				2.3
Pay for private care				9.9				9.2

Source: Author's analysis of Health Survey of England data provided by NatCen Social research 2023

APPENDIX C

Stories of lived experience

This collection of interview material and public presentations about the role of carers serves to illustrate some of the issues elsewhere in the book. Three accounts of 'well networked' individuals show both the importance and limitations of friendship networks, especially for those with insufficient support from relatives, plus some unmet needs for more flexible care services and digital support, and some battles with the National Health Service. Burçu's speech highlights the special difficulties of someone called upon to become a carer at a very young age, perhaps not untypical in London's many migrant communities. Jo and others in the YouTube video made by End Social Care Disgrace show the extraordinary load faced by some older carers of disabled daughters or sons.

The author's previous research in 2011–12 (Gray, 2015) illustrates two important dimensions of community solidarity:

- the potential for mutual aid between seniors where people of mixed levels of dependency, some 'younger old' as well as 'older old', live in close proximity and are brought together in a 'closed' community with some shared social activities, as in many retirement housing schemes;
- the important role of younger volunteers to help mobility-impaired seniors go out and maintain contacts with clubs and activities they used to have.

Names are pseudonyms, except for Jo and Burçu, who were happy to be identified.

Hyacinth is an example of how complex life can be at 87. She chose to move to a 'housing with care' block which has beautiful flats, but in her view the 'care' aspect is never what she really wants. Staff make 15-minute visits to empty bins, sometimes wash dishes, change sheets or tidy up. They did her food shopping when she pressed them after hospital discharge. But she lacks help with deep cleaning or moving furniture, organising paperwork or making medical appointments, except from friends. These things are a big headache for her. During lockdown when visitors were barred she desperately wanted someone to connect her new tablet to broadband, but staff did not help with this – she's not even sure if they knew how. Sometimes she just wants a cup of tea in bed, but it would mean an extra charge even if she asks the carer just to do that and skip the usual things. Hyacinth has many health problems that cause her much pain and loss of sleep. She has huge difficulty getting doctors' appointments and managing her many hospital communications; often she doesn't get enough information, or it arrives very late in the day. Hours on phone lines to hospitals or her doctor eat up her day, often without getting what she feels she needs. It might be easier online, but she doesn't feel able to manage that – her computer and tablet sit in a corner and her new mobile phone doesn't seem to do all the things she wants from it. She misses family support; her son is disabled, and of her three daughters, two live abroad and one over 100 miles away. When busy and in company she is happier and tends to forget her pain, even though it is a very real physical issue. She attends several social clubs when she can, and loves dressing up in her elegant and original clothes. She still does a lot for her church and for the housing-block community on festival days; she delights in making table decorations and pretty lights in bottles.

Elfrida, aged 86, has amazing support from friends and neighbours. She has lived for over 20 years in the same humble back street, partly owner-occupied, partly council housing. She hit a crisis when first her husband died, then she needed an operation at the same time as moving house. Her daughters just couldn't take more time off. Fortunately, friends and neighbours stepped into the breach. Important possessions including her TV were still in the old house; her TV aerial and broadband were yet to be fixed up. Neighbours who had already helped a lot during her bereavement rallied around for moving furniture, shopping and cooking. Uncertain of how much anyone could help, she had to battle with the hospital to grant her a visiting carer during her six-week recovery period, even though she was living alone and could not walk for several days. Later, she found a very helpful cleaner, a refugee, through her seniors' club. Elfrida has helped her with housing issues, found her other cleaning jobs, and has also been teaching her English. The cleaner's three children visit and play happily in her house.

Elfrida has made friends with her neighbours over several years. They bring her food when she is unwell. Many children in the street love to visit her. She sometimes helps with their homework; they appreciate her home cooking, and when well she often bakes bread and cakes for other households. As a retired nurse, she is full of wise advice too.

Burçu (Bu) Keser's speech on being an informal carer

(Given at the launch of the Campsbourne Collective's exhibition mentioned in Chapter 5.)

What is Care?
Care is prioritising the needs of someone else over yours, because let's be honest that's what informal carers do!
- It's ensuring they have taken their medications.
- It's making sure they have food and that they have eaten.
- It's asking when they last washed.
- It's checking to see if they need a re-order of their medications.
- It's checking to see that they have clean clothes, a clean bed, a clean home.
- It's checking to see that they are still breathing and that they are alive!
- It's also grieving for the life you wish you had.

So, who is a Carer?
It is you, me, that child over there that doesn't even realise, that young lady who you saw shopping this morning, that middle aged man caring for his partner. A carer can be anyone, whether they know it or not. Being a carer does not discriminate, it affects a diverse range of people from all walks of life. Whether you're rich, poor, somewhere in between …

What would I want for Carers?

I want it not to be expected or a given for family members. I want all carers (informal and formal) to be paid and recognised as employees. I want carers to receive support, be it emotional, physical, financial as well as support groups and regular retreats to be provided.

Jo's story

The right that would make my life so much better would be the right to a succession for my daughter's care when I'm no longer able to provide it. … I'm aware of my creeping old age, and I want to train up a team to take over from me and look after S. where she wants to be looked after, in her home here, as long as she wants it. At the moment that's not a possibility – continuing care support is only provided year on year, not for the foreseeable future. … Her complex care requires professional staff who understand her individual needs. They need to be trained, so that they can go on to organically train others. As a person needing 24/7 nursing care, and we her unpaid carers, she should have access to this as a right. My living nightmare would then end, and I will be able to die at least knowing that she'll be properly cared for as well if not better than I have done.[1]

Mutual aid in sheltered housing schemes

The following extracts, from notes of interviews and focus groups the author did in sheltered housing schemes during 2011–13, help to illustrate the potential of help between neighbours, while also highlighting some limits where more formal services were

---

[1] Abridged transcript of Jo's part in a video in which several older carers tell their personal history, made by End Social Care Disgrace in November 2023, https://youtu.be/hSGVYEmf6IY?list=PL7427DlyjNCj6r59X_14UT10fQd5reiPv

needed, and the valuable role that younger volunteers could play with mobility issues. (Names of people and housing schemes have been changed.)

James, in a sheltered housing scheme in Colchester

> [We help each other] when someone is discharged from hospital and has no family. Discharge may be very sudden. You've got the weekend and nothing laid on for them. No food in the flat, no one to get prescriptions. In a place like this news goes around, people need help and they get it. If it was not for that people would be stuck.

Focus group at Stonebury Court, a retirement housing estate in Surrey

Susan: I give help to a neighbour aged 97 who has few near relations. Up to a year ago she was very independent. Now her legs have gone and she pays for a cleaner. She sometimes runs out of bread or milk. I give her some. No, I don't mean I go shopping for her. I just give her some for free.

Arthur: I drive Iris to the doctor's. Also to go shopping. If I need things doing there is a man who lives near me who is good at carpentry and moving heavy things.
[Arthur and Sarah both mention that they give people lifts to the station.]
...

Bill: I have done shopping for someone and taken her to the doctor's, but she won't *ask*.

Sarah: When there was snow, someone with a 4 by 4 vehicle helped out – he asked others if they wanted shopping.

Arthur: I give people lifts to the station sometimes. But I don't feel safe driving in snow, I couldn't get to lodge meetings in winter if it wasn't for other members giving me lifts. My grandchildren don't

	even ask me if I want shopping – I had more friends when I lived in Devon.
Jessie:	You need a balance in the community, between those who are able and those who are not. For example, Alice and Colin are frightened to go out in case something happens to [their neighbour] Deirdre – that's not fair, it's a burden on them.
Susan:	If someone wants help here we give it, you don't sit back.
Jessie:	But it's almost like Alice and Colin are Deirdre's carers. Alice is really worried now – she doesn't mind, but now she is bearing a burden.
Arthur:	I had a blackout twice; Matthew helped once, you, Maisie, helped me another time. Once my wife was there. Some people don't like asking for help.
Susan:	The pendant system doesn't always work. I know someone who fell and his pendant was jammed behind his back and he couldn't use it.
Arthur:	As good neighbours we should be aware when things go wrong.
Bill:	I know my neighbour is unwell if she doesn't open the windows in the morning. You have to get to know people's little habits.

Focus group at Marshall Gardens, a sheltered housing scheme in North-west London

David:	Most of the other tenants shop for each other, certainly those that have been here five years or more.
Katie:	There's a lady who doesn't go out. Now she's 91. I visit her about two hours a week. She is depressed. She doesn't want to get dressed. [Madeleine leaves the discussion early to help a neighbour who has had an accident, has her leg in a cast, and needs help with form-filling for the hospital.]

Appendix C

John (with wheelchair): People do my shopping. I also do internet shopping ... when I had a new phone put in, R fixed the cables for me. And he shops for me.

Younger volunteers needed for help with mobility

The wheelchair people: focus group in a sheltered housing scheme in South London

Pat (suffering from Parkinson's Disease): The hospital have now provided me with a wheelchair, which is coming this week. [Pat is almost in tears describing the problems she will face as she becomes chairbound.] The estate manager won't help push a wheelchair. Nor even to go out onto my patio. I would have to pay £8 an hour to get an organisation to come and help me.
Anna: If I'm here I will do it.
Pat: I wouldn't bother you.
Anna: Everyone needs help sometimes. [Later staff comment: Estate managers are not usually supposed to push wheelchairs for residents because this is an insurance/liability issue. But they can put residents in touch with carers and many voluntary services.]

Sheila, interviewed in a sheltered housing scheme in Harlow

Sheila, aged 89, is concerned about her increasing lack of mobility. She would like to mix more with 'the community' (outside the sheltered housing complex) but it's hard to get out − taxis are very costly, even though there is a local discount club for older and disabled people. Sheila used to do play readings with a church women's group of which she was treasurer, but she can't get there now (it's only a few hundred yards away; could no one drive her there?). She doesn't know of anyone. She says of her neighbours: 'A lot of sadness here' – they don't talk much – you can't get much out of them (a reference to the increasing incidence of dementia).

References

Note: all web sites mentioned have been checked as still correct during August 2024.

Adam, S. and Waters, T. (2018) *Options for Raising Taxes.* London: Institute of Fiscal Studies. https://ifs.org.uk/books/options-raising-taxes

ADASS (Association of Directors of Adult Social Services) (2016) *Budget Survey, 2016.* https://www.adass.org.uk/adass-budget-survey-2016-full-report

ADASS (Association of Directors of Adult Social Services) (2022a) *ADASS Spring Survey 2022.*

ADASS (Association of Directors of Adult Social Services) (2022b) *ADASS Survey 2022: Waiting for Care and Support.* https://www.adass.org.uk/documents/adass-survey-2022-waiting-for-care-and-support/

ADASS (Association of Directors of Adult Social Services) (2024) *ADASS Spring Surveys 2024.*

Advani, A., Hughson, H., Summers, A. and Tarrant, H. (2021) *Fixing National Insurance: A Better Way to Fund Social Care.* CAGE Policy Briefing No. 33. Warwick: The University of Warwick. https://warwick.ac.uk/fac/soc/economics/research/centres/cage/publications/policybriefings/2021/fixing_national_insurance_a_better_way_to_fund_social_care/

Age UK (2018) *All the Lonely People: Loneliness in Later Life.* London: Age UK. https://www.ageuk.org.uk/our-impact/policy-research/loneliness-research-and-resources/

Age UK (2023) *The State of Health and Care of Older People, 2023.* London: Age UK. https://www.ageuk.org.uk/globalassets/age-uk/documents/reports-and-publications/reports-and-briefings/health--wellbeing/age-uk-briefing-state-of-health-and-care-july-2023-abridged-version.pdf

Age UK (2024a) *Loneliness, Depression and Anxiety: Exploring the Connection to Mental Health*. London: Age UK. https://www.ageuk.org.uk/our-impact/policy-research/loneliness-research-and-resources/loneliness-depression-and-anxiety-exploring-the-connection-to-mental-health/

Age UK (2024b) *Offline and Overlooked: Digital Exclusion and Its Impact on Older People*. London: Age UK. https://www.ageuk.org.uk/globalassets/age-uk/documents/reports-and-publications/reports-and-briefings/offline-and-overlooked-report.pdf

Alderwick, H., Tallack, C. and Watt, T. (2019) *What Should Be Done to Fix the Crisis in Social Care? Five Priorities for Government*. https://www.health.org.uk/publications/long-reads/what-should-be-done-to-fix-the-crisis-in-social-care (referred to in the text as NEF/WBG for short).

Alderwick, H., Allen, L., Sameen, H., Stevenson, G. and Tallack, C. (2024) *Social Care Funding Reform in England: Choices for the Next Government*. London: Health Foundation. https://www.health.org.uk/publications/long-reads/social-care-funding-reform-in-england

Aldridge, H. and Hughes, F. (2016) *Informal Carers and Poverty in the UK: An Analysis of the Family Resources Survey*. London: New Policy Institute.

Allen, L. (2022) *Poverty and Deprivation amongst Residential Care Workers*. London: Health Foundation. https://www.health.org.uk/sites/default/files/pdf/2022-10/2022%2520-%2520The%2520cost%2520of%2520caring.pdf

Asthana, A. (2017) 'Take care of your elderly mothers and fathers, says Tory minister', *The Guardian*, 31 January. https://www.theguardian.com/society/2017/jan/31/take-care-of-your-elderly-mothers-and-fathers-says-tory-minister

Avlund, K., Lund, R., Holstein, B.E., Due, P., Sakari-Rantala, R. and Heikkinen, R.-L. (2004) 'The impact of structural and functional characteristics of social relations as determinants of functional decline', *The Journals of Gerontology: Series B*, 59(1): S44–S51. https://doi.org/10.1093/geronb/59.1.S44

Banks, J., Batty, G.D., Breedvelt, J., Coughlin, K., Crawford, R., Marmot, M., et al (2024) *English Longitudinal Study of Ageing: Waves 0–10, 1998–2023* [data collection]. 40th edition. UK Data Service. SN: 5050. http://doi.org/10.5255/UKDA-SN-5050-27

References

Beck, D. and Purcell, R. (2013) *International Community Organising*. Bristol: Policy Press. https://doi.org/10.1332/policypress/9781847429773.001.0001

Bedford, S. and Phagoora, J. (2020) *Community Micro-Enterprise as a Driver of Local Economic Development in Social Care*. London: New Economics Foundation. https://neweconomics.org/uploads/files/Community-micro-enterprise2.pdf

Bedford, S. and Button, D. (2022) *Universal Quality Social Care; Transforming Adult Social Care in England*. London: New Economics Foundation with Women's Budget Group. https://neweconomics.org/2022/02/universal-quality-social-care (referred to in the text as NEF/WBG for short).

Bell, D. (2018) 'Free personal care: what the Scottish approach to social care would cost in England', *Health Foundation Newsletter*. https://www.health.org.uk/newsletter-feature/free-personal-care-what-the-scottish-approach-to-social-care-would-cost-in

Bell, D., Bowes, A. and Dawson, A. (2007a) *Free Personal Care in Scotland: Recent Developments: An Examination of the Operation of the Free Personal Care Policy in Scotland: Its Impact, Problems and Limitations*. York: Joseph Rowntree Foundation.

Bell, D., Bowes, A. and Heitmueller, A. (2007b) *Did the Introduction of Free Personal Care in Scotland Result in a Reduction of Informal Care?* St. Gallen: World Demographic Association/University of St. Gallen. https://papers.ssrn.com/sol3/papers.cfm?abstract_id=1884071

Benton, E. and Power, A. (2021) 'Community responses to the coronavirus pandemic: how mutual aid can help', *LSE Public Policy Review*, 1(3). http://eprints.lse.ac.uk/108972/

Beresford, B. and Carr, S. (2012) *Social Care, Service Users and User Involvement*. London: Jessica Kingsley.

Bimpson, E., Dayson, C., Ellis-Paine, A., Gilbertson, J., Kara, H. and Leather, D. (2023) *Evaluation of the Leeds Neighbourhood Networks*. London: Centre for Ageing Better. https://shura.shu.ac.uk/31870/1/Neighbourhood-networks-model-for-community-based-support.pdf

Blair, T. (1998) *The Third Way*. London: Fabian Society.

Blood, I. and Pannell, J. (2012) *Supported Housing for Older People in the UK: An Evidence Review*. York: Joseph Rowntree Foundation.

Boneham, M. and Sixsmith, J. (2006) 'The voices of older women in a disadvantaged community: issues of health and social capital', *Social Science and Medicine*, 62(2): 269–79.

Bonsang, E. (2009) 'Does informal care from children to their elderly parents substitute for formal care in Europe?', *Journal of Health Economics*, 28: 143–154.

Booth, R. (2023) 'UK care home bosses demand next government funds 44% pay rise for staff', *The Guardian*, 19 September. https://www.theguardian.com/society/2023/sep/19/uk-care-home-bosses-demand-next-government-funds-44-pay-rise-for-staff

Bovaird, T. and Willis, M. (2012) 'Commissioning for quality and outcomes', in Glasby, J. (ed) *Commissioning for Health and Wellbeing*. Bristol: Bristol University Press, chapter 7, pp 145–65.

Bowes, A., Dawson, A. and Ashworth, R. (2019) 'Time for care: exploring time use by carers of older people', *Ageing and Society*: 1–24. Doi:10.1017/S0144686X19000205.

Boyle, D. and Bird, S. (2014) *Give and Take: How Timebanking is Transforming Healthcare*. Stroud: Timebanking UK.

Brimblecombe, N., Pickard, L., King, D. and Knapp, M. (2017) 'Barriers to receipt of social care services for working carers and the people they care for in times of austerity', *Journal of Social Policy*, 47(2): 215–33.

Brimblecombe, N., Fernandez, J.L., Knapp, M., Rehil, A. and Wittenberg, R. (2018) *Unpaid Care in England: Future Patterns and Potential Support Strategies*. London: London School of Economics, PSSRU.

Buckner, L.J. (2017) *Caring More Than Most*. London: Contact. https://contact.org.uk/wp-content/uploads/2021/03/caring_more_than_most_full_report.pdf

Burgess, G. (2014) *Evaluation of the Cambridgeshire Timebanks*. Cambridge: Cambridge University, Cambridge Centre for Housing and Planning Research, Department of Land Economy.

Cahn, E.S. and Gray, C. (2011) 'Co-production from a normative perspective', in Pestoff, V., Brandsen, T. and Verschuere, B. (eds) *New Public Governance, the Third Sector and Co-production*. Abingdon: Routledge, chapter 7, pp 114–38.

Cahn, E. and Gray, C. (2015) 'The time bank solution', *Stanford Social Innovation Review*, Summer. https://timebanking.org

References

Cahn, E. and Gray, C. (2021) *The Other Pandemic: Social Isolation and Timebanking*. New Weather Institute. Steyning, Sussex: Real Press. www.newweather.org/www.therealpress.co.uk

Callaghan, L., Netten, A., Darton, R., Bäumker, T. and Holder, J. (2008) *Social Well-Being in Extra Care Housing: Emerging Themes, Interim Report*. York: Joseph Rowntree Foundation. http://www.pssru.ac.uk/pdf/dp2524_2.pdf

Cambridge Centre for Housing and Planning Research (2014) *Evaluation of the Cambridgeshire Timebanks*. Cambridge: Cambridge University, Department of Land Economy. https://www.cchpr.landecon.cam.ac.uk/Research/Start-Year/2012/Evaluation-Cambridgeshire-Timebanking-project/Final_Project

Cambridgeshire County Council (2019) *Neighbourhood Cares Pilot, Final Report*. Cambridge: Cambridgeshire County Council. https://www.buurtzorg.org.uk/wp-content/uploads/2018/11/Neighbourhood-Cares-Report-NCP.pdf

Cameron, A.M., Johnson, E.K., Willis, P.B., Lloyd, L.E. and Smith, R.C. (2020) 'Exploring the role of volunteers in social care for older adults', *Quality in Ageing and Older Adults*, 21(2): 129–39. https://doi.org/10.1108/QAOA-02-2020-0005

Campbell, D. (2019) '84% of care home beds in England owned by private firms', *The Guardian*, 19 September. https://www.theguardian.com/society/2019/sep/19/84-of-care-home-beds-in-england-owned-by-private-firms

Cantillon, S. and O'Toole, F. (2022) 'Citizens' basic income in Scotland: on the road to somewhere', *European Journal of Social Security*, 24(3): 230–42. https://doi.org/10.1177/13882627221114373

Care Management Matters (2023) 'ADASS spring survey', 21 June. https://www.caremanagementmatters.co.uk/adass-spring-survey-2023/

Carers UK (2019) *State of Caring*. London: Carers UK. https://www.carersuk.org/reports/state-of-caring-2019/

Carers UK (2020a) *Carers Week 2020 Research Report*. London: Carers UK. https://www.carersuk.org/reports/carers-week-2020-research-report/

Carers UK (2020b) *Unseen and Under-valued*. London: Carers UK. https://www.carersuk.org/reports/unseen-and-undervalued-the-value-of-unpaid-care-provided-to-date-during-the-covid-19-pandemic/

Carers UK (2021) *Valuing Carers 2021*. London: Carers UK. https://www.carersuk.org/media/2d5le03c/valuing-carers-report.pdf

Carers UK (2022) *The State of Caring 2022*. London: Carers UK. https://www.carersuk.org/media/ew5e4swg/cuk_state_of_caring_2022_report.pdf

Carers UK (2023a) *Carers' Employment Rights Today, Tomorrow and in the Future*. London: Carers UK. https://www.carersuk.org/policy-and-research/state-of-caring-survey/

Carers UK (2023b) *The Impact of Caring on Finances*. London: Carers UK. https://www.carersuk.org/reports/state-of-caring-survey-2023-the-impact-of-caring-on-finances/

Carers UK (2023c) *The State of Caring 2023*. London: Carers UK. https://www.carersuk.org/media/xgwlj0gn/soc23-health-report_web.pdf

Carey, H., Chandler, J. and Steadman, K. (2018) *Who Cares? The Implications of Informal Care and Work for Policymakers and Employers*. London: Work Foundation. https://www.lancaster.ac.uk/work-foundation/publications/who-cares/

Carmichael, F., Charles, S. and Hulme, C. (2010) 'Who will care? Employment participation and willingness to supply informal care', *Journal of Health Economics*, 29: 182–190.

Carrino, L., Glaser, K. and Avendono, M. (2020) 'Later retirement, job strain, and health: evidence from the new state pension age in the United Kingdom', *Health Economics*, 29(8): 849–954.

Cattan, M., White, M., Bond, J. and Learmouth, A. (2005) 'Preventing social isolation and loneliness among older people: a systematic review of health promotion interventions', *Ageing and Society*, 25(1): 41–67. https://doi.org/10.1017/S0144686X04002594

Cattell, V. (2001) 'Poor people, poor places, and poor health: the mediating role of social networks and social capital', *Social Science and Medicine*, 52(10): 1501–16.

Cavendish, C. (2022) *Social Care: Independent Report*. London: HM Government Publishing Service. https://assets.publishing.service.gov.uk/media/6228f5f3e90e0747a30ca996/social-care-reform-Baroness-Cavendish-report.pdf

Central Bedfordshire Council (nd) *Community Catalysts Case Studies: Community Microenterprise*. Bedford; Central Bedfordshire Council. https://www.centralbedfordshire.gov.uk/info/22/information_for_professionals/332/community_micro-enterprise/2

References

Centre for Ageing Better (2020) *Ever More Needed: The Role of the Leeds Neighbourhood Networks during the COVID-19 Pandemic.* London: Centre for Ageing Better. https://ageing-better.org.uk/resources/ever-more-needed-role-leeds-neighbourhood-networks-during-covid-19-pandemic

Centre for Ageing Better (2022) *Context: The State of Ageing 2022.* London: Centre for Ageing Better. https://ageing-better.org.uk/context-state-ageing-2022

Centre for Ageing Better (2023) *Neighbourhood Networks: A Model for Community-based Support.* London: Centre for Ageing Better. https://ageing-better.org.uk/neighbourhood-networks-model-community-based-su ort-web-version

Centre for Ageing Better (nd) *What's an Age-friendly Community?* https://ageing-better.org.uk/age-friendly-communities/eight-domains

Chan, T. and Ermisch, J. (2015) 'Proximity of couples to parents: influences of gender, labor market, and family', *Demography*, 52(2): 379–99.

Chappell, N. and Blandford, A. (1991) 'Informal and formal care: exploring the complementarity', *Ageing and Society*, 11(4): 299–317.

Chatzidikis, A., Hakim, J., Littler, J., Rottenberg, C. and Segal, L. (The Care Collective) (2020) *The Care Manifesto.* London: Verso.

Chevée, A. (2022) 'Mutual aid in north London during the Covid-19 pandemic', *Social Movement Studies*, 21(4): 413–19. Doi: 10.1080/14742837.2021.1890574.

Clement, N., Holbrook, A., Forster, D., Macneil, J., Smith, M., Lyons, K., et al (2017) 'Time-banking, co-production and normative principles: putting normative principles into practice', *International Journal of Community Currency Research*, 21: 36–52. http://www.ijccr.net

Cobham, A. and Janský, P. (2020) *Estimating Illicit Financial Flows: A Critical Guide to the Data, Methodologies, and Findings.* Oxford: Oxford Academic. https://doi.org/10.1093/oso/9780198854418.003.0005

Cocking, C., Drury, J., McTague, M. and Perach, R. (2023) 'Can group-based strategies increase community resilience? Longitudinal predictors of sustained participation in Covid-19 mutual aid and community support groups', *Journal of Allied Social Psychology*, 53(11): 1059–75. https://doi.org/10.1111/jasp.12995

Comas-Herrera, A., Darton, R., King, D., Malley, J., Pickard, L. and Wittenberg, R. (2006) *Future Demand for Long-Term Care, 2002 to 2041: Projections of Demand for Long-Term Care for Older People in England*. PSSRU Discussion Paper 2330. London: London School of Economics. https://www.pssru.ac.uk/pdf/dp2330.pdf

Competition and Markets Authority (2017) *Care Homes Market Study: Final Report*. London: Competition and Markets Authority. https://assets.publishing.service.gov.uk/media/5a1fdf30e5274a750b82533a/care-homes-market-study-final-report.pdf

Corlett, A. (2018) *Passing On: Options for Reforming Inheritance Taxation*. London: Resolution Foundation. https://www.resolutionfoundation.org/publications/passing-on-options-for-reforming-inheritance-taxation/

Cottam, H. (2019) *Radical Help: How We Can Remake the Relationships Between Us and Revolutionise the Welfare State*. London: Virago.

Crawford, R. and Stoye, G. (2017) *The Prevalence and Dynamics of Social Care Receipt*. London: Institute for Fiscal Studies.

Croucher, K., Hicks, L. and Jackson, K. (2006) *Housing with Care for Later Life: A Literature Review*. York: Joseph Rowntree Foundation.

Cunyoen, K., Bailiang, W., Emiko, T., Tanaka, T., Watanabe, K.W. and Watanabe, W. (2016) 'Association between a change in social interaction and dementia among elderly people', *International Journal of Gerontology*, 10(2): 76–80. https://doi.org/10.1016/j.ijge.2016.03.006

Cushman, M. and Millbourne, L. (2015) 'Complying, transforming or resisting in the new austerity? Realigning social welfare and independent action among English voluntary organisations', *Journal of Social Policy*, 44(3): 463–85. Doi:10.1017/S0047279414000853.

References

Darton, R., Bäumker, T., Callaghan, L., Holder, J., Netten, A. and Towers, A. (2008) *Evaluation of the Extra Care Housing Funding Initiative: Initial Report*. PSSRU Discussion Paper 2506/2. Canterbury: University of Kent, Personal and Social Services Research Unit. http://www.pssru.ac.uk/project-pages/extra-care-housing/index.php#reports

Davis, N., Campbell, L. and McNulty, C. (2019) *How to Fix the Funding of Social Care*. London: Institute for Government.

Dayan, M. (2023) *Time to Worry about the Social Care Squeeze*. London: Nuffield Trust [online blog]. https://www.nuffieldtrust.org.uk/news-item/time-to-worry-about-the-social-care-squeeze

Dayson, C., Gilbertson, J., Chambers, J., Ellis-Paine, A. and Kara, H. (2022) *How Community Organisations Contribute to Healthy Ageing: Evidence from the Evaluation of the Leeds Neighbourhood Networks*. London: Centre for Ageing Better. https://ageing-better.org.uk/resources/leeds-neighbourhood-network-phase-two

Degavre, F. and Nyssens, M. (2014) 'European care regimes in a context of deep transformation under a Polanyian approach: what possible roles for social enterprises?', *Secteur non marchand, milieux associatifs, organismes communautaires: des mondes en recomposition*. https://dial.uclouvain.be/pr/boreal/object/boreal:154308

Demos (2023) *The Triple Dividend of Home Improvement*. London: Demos. https://demos.co.uk/wp-content/uploads/2023/11/Triple-Dividend-Part-Three.pdf

Department of Health (2014) *Care and Support Statutory Guidance Issued under the Care Act 2014*. https://assets.publishing.service.gov.uk/media/5a7dcf2aed915d2ac884dafa/Care-Act-Guidance.pdf

Department of Health and Social Care (2024) *Care and Support Statutory Guidance*, para. 10.26. https://www.gov.uk/government/publications/care-act-statutory-guidance/care-and-support-statutory-guidance#using-the-care-act-guidance

Department of Health and Social Care, Cabinet Office and Office of the Prime Minister (2022) *Adult Social Care Charging Reform, Further Details*. London: UK Government. https://www.gov.uk/government/publications/build-back-better-our-plan-for-health-and-social-care/adult-social-care-charging-reform-further-details

Derbyshire County Council (2013) *Public Health Investment to Increase Accessibility of Affordable Warmth Interventions to the Most Vulnerable Populations*. Derby: Derbyshire County Council. https://www.derbyshirepartnership.gov.uk/anti-poverty-strategy/fuel-poverty-and-affordable-warmth/fuel-poverty-and-affordable-warmth.aspx

Dodsworth, E. and Oung, C. (2023) 'How much social care does each country fund?', in *Adult Social Care in the Four Countries of the UK*. London: Nuffield Trust.

Dolan, P., Krekel, C., Shreedhar, G., Lee, H., Marshall, C. and Smith, A. (2021) *Happy to Help: The Welfare Effects of a Nationwide Micro-volunteering Programme*. London: London School of Economics, Centre for Economic Performance. http://cep.lse.ac.uk/pubs/download/dp1772.pdf

Dowling, E. (2021) *The Care Crisis: What Caused It and How Can We End It?* London: Verso.

DPAC (Disabled People Against Cuts) (2019) *UBI: Solution or Illusion*. https://dpac.uk.net/2019/01/universal-basic-income/

Dubb, S. (2022) 'Edgar Cahn's second act: timebanking and the return of mutual aid', *Non-profit Quarterly*, 9 February. https://nonprofitquarterly.org/edgar-cahns-second-act-time-banking-and-the-return-of-mutual-aid/

Dunatchik, A., Icardi, R., Roberts, C. and Blake, M. (2016) *Predicting Unmet Social Care Needs and Links with Well-being: Findings from the Secondary Analysis*. London: NatCen Social Research.

Espiet-Kilty, R. (2016) 'David Cameron, citizenship and the big society: a new social model?', *Revue Française de Civilisation Britannique*, 21(1). http://journals.openedition.org/rfcb/796

Feeley, D. (2021) *Independent Review of Adult Social Care in Scotland*. Edinburgh: Scottish Government. https://tinyurl.com/ymwpkvte

Felici, M. (2020) *Social Capital and the Response to Covid-19*. Cambridge: Cambridge University, Bennett Institute for Public Policy. https://www.bennettinstitute.cam.ac.uk/blog/social-capital-and-response-covid-19/

Fihel, A., Kalbarczyk, M. and Nicińska, A. (2022) Childlessness, geographical proximity and non-family support in 12 European countries. *Ageing and Society*, 42(11): 2695–720. Doi:10.1017/S0144686X21000313.

References

Fiori, K.L., Antonucci, T.C. and Akiyama, H. (2018) 'Profiles of social relations amongst older adults: a multi-dimensional approach', *Journals of Gerontology: Psychological Sciences*, 61: 25–32.

Fraser of Allender Institute (2022) *Social Care Reform in Scotland: Context, Costs and Questions*. Glasgow: University of Strathclyde Business School.

Frericks, P., Jensen, P.H. and Pfau-Effinger, B. (2014) 'Social rights and employment rights related to family care: family care regimes in Europe', *Journal of Aging Studies*, 29: 66–77.

FRS (Family Resources Survey) (2018) and reports and published data files from other years. https://assets.publishing.service.gov.uk/media/5e78aabfe90e073e369427ac/family-resources-survey-2018-19.pdf

Gostoli, U. and Silverman, E. (2019) 'Modelling social care provision in an agent-based framework with kinship networks', *Royal Society Open Science*, 6: Article 190029. https://doi.org/10.1098/rsos.190029

Gray, A. (2006) *Growing Old in a London Borough*. London: Families and Social Capital Group, London South Bank University. https://www.lsbu.ac.uk%2F__data%2Fassets%2Fpdf_file%2F0004%2F9382%2Fgrowing-old-london-families-research-working-paper.pdf

Gray, A. (2009) 'The social capital of older people', *Ageing and Society*, 29(1): 5–31.

Gray, A. (2015) 'Social capital and neighbourhood in older people's housing', in Nyqvist, F. and Forsman, A. (eds) *Social Capital as a Health Resource in Later Life: The Relevance of Context*. New York: Springer, pp 65–88.

Gray, A. and Worlledge, G. (2018) 'Addressing loneliness and isolation in retirement housing', *Ageing and Society*, 38(1): 615–44. Doi: 10.1017/S0144686X16001239.

Greater Manchester Combined Authority (2021) *Framework for Creating Age-Friendly Homes in Greater Manchester, 2021–2024*. Manchester: Greater Manchester Combined Authority. https://www.greatermanchester-ca.gov.uk/what-we-do/ageing/creating-age-friendly-homes-in-greater-manchester/

Hall, K. (2022) *Can Social Enterprises Tackle the Social Care Crisis?* University of Birmingham, Social Sciences Blog, 8 November. https://blog.bham.ac.uk/socialsciencesbirmingham/2022/11/08/can-social-enterprises-tackle-the-social-care-crisis/

Hall, K. and Alexander, C. (2023) 'Exploring the distinctiveness of social enterprises delivering adult social care in England', *Health and Social Care in the Community*, 2023. Article ID 9454428, https://onlinelibrary.wiley.com/doi/10.1155/2023/9454428

Hamblin, K., Heyes, J. and Fast, J. (eds) (2024) *Combining Work and Care: Carer Leave and Related Employment Policies in International Context*. Bristol: Policy Press. https://bristoluniversitypressdigital.com/edcollbook-oa/book/9781447365723/9781447365723.xml

Hanover Housing Group (2009) *Hanover Inpractice: 1, September, Sect. 5*.

Harrop, A. and Cooper, B. (2023) *A National Care Service for All*. London: Fabian Society. https://fabians.org.uk/a-national-care-service-for-all/

Hayashi, M. (2012) 'Japan's Fureai Kippu Timebanking in elderly care: origins, development challenges and impact', *International Journal of Community Currency Research*, 16(A): 30–44. https://doi.org/10.1111/hsc.13166

Healthcare Improvement Scotland (2019) *Learning from Neighbourhood Care Test Sites in Scotland*. Edinburgh: NHS Scotland. https://ihub.scot/media/6937/20191205-neighbourhood-care-eval-eevit-v014final.pdf

Health Foundation (2018) *Social Care Funding Options: How Much and Where From?* London: Health Foundation. https://reader.health.org.uk/social-care-funding-options

Health Foundation (2023) *Adult Social Care Funding Pressures*. London: Health Foundation. https://www.health.org.uk/publications/long-reads/adult-social-care-funding-pressures and Technical Annex on https://www.health.org.uk/sites/default/files/2023-09/ASC%2520Funding%2520Pressures%2520Model%25202023%2520update%2520-%2520TECHNICAL%2520ANNEX.pdf

Health Foundation (2024) *Social Care Funding Reform*. London: Health Foundation. https://www.health.org.uk/publications/long-reads/social-care-funding-reform-in-england

Health Survey of England (2017, published 2018) *Annual Published Report*. NHS Digital. https://digital.nhs.uk/data-and-information/publications/statistical/health-survey-for-england/2017#highlights

References

Health Survey of England (2021) *Annual Published Report*. NHS Digital. https://digital.nhs.uk/data-and-information/publications/statistical/health-survey-for-england/2021

Hemingway, H. and Marmot, M. (1999) 'Evidence-based cardiology: psychosocial factors in the etiology and prognosis of coronary artery disease. Systemic review of prospective cohort studies', *British Medical Journal*, 318: 1460–7. https://www.bmj.com/content/318/7196/1460

Hirst, M. (2002) 'Trends in informal care in Great Britain during the 1990s', *Health and Social Care in the Community*, 9(6): 348–57. https://doi.org/10.1046/j.0966-0410.2001.00313.x

Hirst, M.A. (2005) 'Estimating the prevalence of unpaid adult care over time', *Research, Policy and Planning*, 23(1): 1–16. http://ssrg.org.uk/research-policy-and-planning-volume-23/

HMRC (His Majesty's Revenue and Customs) (2023) *Multinational Top-up Tax and Domestic top-up Tax: UK Adoption of OECD Pillar 2*. London: HMRC. https://www.gov.uk/government/publications/introduction-of-the-new-multinational-top-up-tax-and-domestic-top-up-tax/multinational-top-up-tax-and-domestic-top-up-tax-uk-adoption-of-oecd-pillar-2#summary-of-impacts

Holmes, J. (2016) *An Overview of the Domiciliary Care Market in the UK*. Wellington: UK Home Care Association.

Holtham, G. (2018) *Paying for Social Care*. Cardiff: Welsh Government. https://www.gov.wales/written-statement-paying-social-care-independent-report-professor-gerald-holtham

Holt-Lunstad, J., Smith, T.B. and Layton, J.B. (2010) 'Social relationships and mortality risk: a meta-analytic review', *PLOS Medicine*. Doi: 10.1371/journal.pmed.1000316.

House of Commons Library (2022) *Paying for Adult Social Care in England*. SN01911. London: House of Commons. http://commonslibrary.parliament.uk

House of Commons Library Research Briefing (2023) *UK Disability Statistics: Prevalence and Life Experiences*. https://commonslibrary.parliament.uk/research-briefings/cbp-9602/

House of Commons Library Research Briefing (2024) *Who Provides Informal Care?* https://commonslibrary.parliament.uk/research-briefings/cbp-10017/

House of Commons Research (2023) *UK Disability Statistics; Prevalence and Life Experiences*. Briefing no. 09602. London: House of Commons

House of Commons Research (2024) *Higher Education Student Numbers*, Briefing no. 7857. London: House of Commons. https://researchbriefings.files.parliament.uk/documents/CBP-7857/CBP-7857.pdf

House of Lords (2021) *A Gloriously Ordinary Life; Spotlight on Adult Social Care*. Adult Social Care Committee, Report of Session 2022–23. London: House of Lords. https://committees.parliament.uk/publications/31917/documents/193737/default/

Hu, B., Hancock, R. and Wittenberg, R. (2018) *Projections of Demand and Expenditure on Adult Social Care 2015 to 2040*. PSSRU Discussion Paper 2944. London: London School of Economics. https://core.ac.uk/download/pdf/159070032.pdf

Hu, B., Hancock, R. and Wittenberg, R. (2020) *Projections of Demand and Expenditure on Adult Social Care 2018 to 2038*. CPEC Working Paper 7. London: London School of Economics. https://www.lse.ac.uk/cpec/assets/documents/cpec-working-paper-7.pdf

Humphries, R. (2022) *Ending the Social Care Crisis: A New Road to Reform*. Bristol: Bristol University Press.

Idriss, O., Tallack, C., Shembavnekar, N. and Carter, M. (2021) *Social Care Funding Gap: Technical Annex*. London: Health Foundation. https://www.health.org.uk/news-and-comment/charts-and-infographics/REAL-social-care-funding-gap

Iecovitch, E., Jacobs, E. and Stessman, E. (2011) 'Loneliness, social networks, and mortality: 18 years of follow-up', *International Journal of Aging and Human Development*, 72(3): 243–63.

Incisive Health (2019) *Care Deserts: The Impact of a Dysfunctional Market in Adult Social Care Provision: A Report for Age UK*. London: Age UK. https://www.ageuk.org.uk/globalassets/age-uk/documents/reports-and-publications/reports-and-briefings/care--support/care-deserts---age-uk-report.pdf

Independent Age (2020) *Free Personal Care: Insights from Scotland*. London: Independent Age. https://www.independentage.org/sites/default/files/2020-10/Report_Final.pdf

References

Institute for Government (2023) *Performance Tracker 2023: Adult Social Care*. https://www.instituteforgovernment.org.uk/publication/performance-tracker-2023/adult-social-care

Intergenerational Foundation (2023) *Play Fair: Equalising the Taxation of Earned and Unearned Income*. https://www.if.org.uk/research-posts/play-fair-equalising-the-taxation-of-earned-and-unearned-income/

IPPR (Institute for Public Policy Research) (2021) 'Securing a living income in Scotland: towards a minimum income guarantee'. London: IPPR. https://www.ippr.org/articles/what-is-a-minimum-income-guarantee

Ismail, S., Thorlby, R. and Holder, H. (2014) *Focus on Social Care for Older People: Reductions in Adult Social Services for Older People in England*. London: Health Foundation with Nuffield Trust.

James, B.D., Wilson, R.S., Barnes, L.L. and Bennett, D.A. (2011) 'Late-life social activity and cognitive decline in old age', *Journal of the International Neuropsychological Society*, 17(6): 998–1005.

Jisca, S., Kuiper, M.Z., Richard, C., Oude, V., Sytse, U.Z., van den Heuvel, E.R., et al (2015) 'Social relationships and risk of dementia: a systematic review and meta-analysis of longitudinal cohort studies', *Ageing Research Reviews*, 22: 39–57. https://doi.org/10.1016/j.arr.2015.04.006

Jones, M., Beardmore, A., Biddle, M., Gibson, A., Ismail, S.U., McClean, S., et al (2023) 'Apart but not alone? A cross-sectional study of neighbour support in a major UK urban area during the COVID-19 lockdown', *Emerald Open Research*, 2(37). https://doi.org/10.35241/emeraldopenres.13731.1

Karlsberg-Schaffer, S. (2015) 'The effect of free personal care for the elderly on informal caregiving', *Health Economics*, 24(S1): 104–17. http://onlinelibrary.wiley.com/doi/10.1002/hec.3146/abstract

Kartupelis, J. (2021) *Making Relational Care Work for Older People: Exploring Innovation and Best Practice in Everyday Life*. London: Routledge.

Kavada, A. (2022) 'Creating a hyperlocal infrastructure of care: COVID-19 mutual aid groups in the UK', in Bringel, B. and Pleyers, G. (eds) *Social Movements and Politics During COVID-19: Crisis, Solidarity and Change in a Global Pandemic*. Bristol: Bristol University Press, pp 147–54. https://bristoluniversitypressdigital.com/display/book/9781529217254/ch031.xml

Keating, N., Oftinowski, P., Wenger, C., Fast, J. and Derksen, L. (2003) 'Understanding the caring capacity of informal networks of frail seniors: a case for care networks', *Ageing and Society*, 23(1): 115–27. https://doi.org/10.1017/S0144686X02008954

King, D. and Pickard, L. (2013) 'When is a carer's employment at risk? Longitudinal analysis of unpaid care and employment in midlife in England', *Health and Social Care in the Community*, 21(3): 303–14.

King's Fund (2023) *Social Care 360: Expenditure*. London: King's Fund. https://www.kingsfund.org.uk/insight-and-analysis/long-reads/social-care-360-expenditure

King's Fund (2024a) *Social Care 360*. London: King's Fund. https://www.kingsfund.org.uk/insight-and-analysis/long-reads/social-care-360#expenditure-and-providers

King's Fund (2024b) *Social Care in a Nutshell*. London: King's Fund. https://www.kingsfund.org.uk/insight-and-analysis/long-reads/social-care-360-expenditure#4.-expenditure

Kropotkin, P. (2009 [1902]) *Mutual Aid: A Factor of Evolution*. London: Freedom Press.

Leeds City Council (2018) *Commissioning Code of Practice*. Leeds: Leeds City Council. https://democracy.leeds.gov.uk/%2528X%25281%2529S%2528fkn0jfigeevz5oferbjpjk55%2529%2529/documents/s174384/Compact%2520Report%2520Appendix%25202%2520050418.pdf

Lemmon, E. (2020) 'Utilisation of personal care services in Scotland: the influence of unpaid carers', *Journal of Long-Term Care*: 54–69. Doi: 10.31389/jltc.23.

Li, Y., Pickles, A. and Savage, M. (2005) 'Social capital and social trust in Britain', *European Sociological Review*, 21(2): 109–23.

Limbrick, P. (2016) *Caring Activism: A 21st Century Concept of Care*. Clifford: Interconnection.

Litwin, H. and Shiovitz-Ezra, S. (2015) 'Social network type and health among older Americans', Nyqvist, F. and Forsman, A. (eds) *Social Capital as a Health Resource in Later Life: The Relevance of Context*. New York: Springer, pp 15–32.

Lloyd, L. (2023) *Unpaid Care Policies in the UK: Rights, Resources and Relationships*. Bristol: Bristol University Press.

References

Local Government Association (2021) *Case Study: Leeds City Council: Using Neighbourhood Networks to Connect Communities.* https://www.local.gov.uk/case-studies/leeds-city-council-using-neighbourhood-networks-connect-communities, London.

Local Government Association/Department of Health (2015) *Guide to the Care Act 2014 and the Implications for Providers.* https://www.local.gov.uk/sites/default/files/documents/Guidance_on_the_impact_of_the_Care_Act.pdf, London: Department of Health.

Lunt, N. (2019) 'Asset-based and strengths-based community initiatives in the UK', *Global Social Security Review*, 11. https://www.researchgate.net/profile/Neil-Lunt/publication/339376026_Asset-based_and_strengths-based_community_initiatives_in_the_UK/links/613759000360302a0084793f/Asset-based-and-strengths-based-community-initiatives-in-the-UK.pdf

Lyall, S. (2017) *Big Care Providers are Wasting Taxpayers' Money.* New Economics Foundation blog. https://neweconomics.org/2017/03/big-care-providers-wasting-taxpayers-money

Maher, J. and Green, H. (2002) *Carers 2000*. London: The Stationery Office.

Manchester Local Care Organisation (2023) *Better Outcomes, Better Lives.* Manchester: Manchester City Council. https://www.manchesterlco.org/app/uploads/2023/11/Commissioning-Plan-23-24.pdf

Mayo, M. (2022) 'Covid-19 and mutual aid: prefigurative a roaches to caring?', *Concept*, 13(3). http://concept.lib.ed.ac.uk/ Online ISSN 2042-6 968

McNamee, P. (2006) *Effects of Free Personal Care in Scotland.* London: King's Fund. https://archive.kingsfund.org.uk/concern/published_works/000037029%3Flocale%3Dzh

Miller, A. (2019) *Essentials of Basic Income.* Edinburgh: Luath Press.

Morning Star, 18 February 2019, 'ACORN UK; Taking what's ours'. https://www.google.com/url?sa=t&source=web&rct=j&opi=89978449&url=https://morningstaronline.co.uk/article/f/acorn-uk-taking-whats-ours

Murphy, R. (2024) *Taxing Wealth Report* [blog]. https://taxingwealth.uk/2023/09/08/abolishing-the-lower-rate-of-national-insurance-for-high-earning-employees/

Musselwhite, C. (2018) *Age-friendly Transport for Greater Manchester*. Swansea: Swansea University, Centre for Innovative Ageing. https://ageing-better.org.uk/resources/age-friendly-transport-greater-manchester

Nair, V. (2023) 'How is the world tackling tax avoidance by multi-national companies?', *Economic Review*, 41(1). https://ifs.org.uk/articles/how-world-tackling-tax-avoidance-multinational-companies

NAO (National Audit Office) (2021) *The Adult Social Care Market in England*. London: NAO. https://www.nao.org.uk/wp-content/uploads/2021/03/The-adult-social-care-market-in-England.pdfandved=2ahUKEwjMjJHrwJqFAxUpWEEAHREpCHwQFnoECCEQAQ

NatCen Social Research, University College London, Department of Epidemiology and Public Health (2023) *Health Survey for England 7th Release*, UK Data Service. SN: 2000021. Doi: http://doi.org/10.5255/UKDA-Series-2000021 [Data files for 2011 and 2018 were used for this book].

Naughton-Doe, R., Cameron, A. and Carpenter, J. (2021) 'Timebanking and the co-production of preventive social care with adults: what can we learn from the challenges of implementing person-to-person timebanks in England?', *Health and Social Care in the Community*, 29(5): 1280–95.

Neate, R. (2023) 'Modest wealth tax could raise more than £10bn for public services, says TUC', *The Guardian*, 11 August. https://www.theguardian.com/politics/2023/aug/11/modest-wealth-tax-could-raise-more-than-10bn-for-public-services-says-tuc

Needham, C., Allen, K. and Hall, K. (2014) 'Grass roots entrepreneurship and innovation: micro-enterprise in social care'. Paper for International Research Society for Public Management Annual Conference, Ottawa, Canada. https://www.birmingham.ac.uk/documents/college-social-sciences/social-policy/hsmc/publications/2014/irspm-paper-hall-needham-allen-grassroots-panel.pdf

Needham, C., Allen, K. and Hall, K. (2017) *Micro-enterprise and Personalisation*. Bristol: Policy Press.

NEF/WBG; see Bedford and Button (2022).

References

NHS (2023) *NHS Volunteer Responders: Volunteer Survey and Engagement Meeting Results.* https://www.england.nhs.uk/long-read/nhs-volunteer-responders-volunteer-survey-and-engagement-meeting-results/

NHS Digital (2018) *Social Care Survey.* https://digital.nhs.uk/data-and-information/publications/statistical/adult-social-care-activity-and-finance-report/2018-19/2.-requests-for-support

NHS Digital (2019) *Adult Social Care and Finance Report, England, 2018/19.* https://digital.nhs.uk/data-and-information/publications/statistical/adult-social-care-activity-and-finance-report/2018-19#

NHS Digital (2022) *Adult Social Care and Finance Report, England, 2021/22.* https://digital.nhs.uk/data-and-information/publications/statistical/adult-social-care-activity-and-finance-report/2021-22

NHS Digital (2024) *Adult Social Care Statistics in England: An Overview.* https://digital.nhs.uk/data-and-information/publications/statistical/adult-social-care-statistics-in-england/an-overview

NHS with Royal Voluntary Service (2020) *Findings from Volunteers Participating in the NHS Volunteer Responder Programme During Covid-19 – April to August 2020: Working Paper Two.* London: Royal Voluntary Service. https://www.royalvoluntaryservice.org.uk/media/kjdpkebn/working_paper_two_patient_findings_271120.pdf

NHS with Royal Voluntary Service (2021) *Findings from Those Referring into the NHS Volunteer Responder Programme during COVID-19: Working Paper Three.* London: Royal Voluntary Service. https://www.royalvoluntaryservice.org.uk/media/xhvdlf24/nhsvr_working_paper_three_referrer_findings.pdf

NISRA (Northern Ireland Statistics and Research Agency) (2022) *Census 2021 Main Statistics Health, Disability and Unpaid Care Tables.* Belfast: NISRA. https://www.nisra.gov.uk/publications/census-2021-main-statistics-health-disability-and-unpaid-care-tables

Noddings, N. (2013) *Caring: A Relational Approach to Ethics and Moral Education.* 2nd edition. Berkeley and Los Angeles: University of California Press.

Nuffield Trust (2023) *The Decline of Publicly Funded Social Care for Older Adults*. https://www.nuffieldtrust.org.uk/resource/the-decline-of-publicly-funded-social-care-for-older-adults

Nyqvist, F. and Forsman, A. (eds) (2015) Editors' Introduction, in Nyqvist, F. and Forsman, A. (eds) *Social Capital as a Health Resource in Later Life: The Relevance of Context*. New York: Springer, pp 1–14.

O'Dwyer, E., Beascochea-Segui, N. and Souza, L.G.S. (2021) 'Rehearsing post-Covid-19 citizenship: social representations of UK Covid-19 mutual aid', *British Journal of Social Psychology*, 61: 1245–62.

OECD (Organization for Economic Co-operation and Development) (2020) *PF2.3: Additional Leave Entitlements for Working Parents*. Paris: OECD. https://www.oecd.org/els/soc/PF2_3_Additional_leave_entitlements_of_workingparents.pdf

Office for Health Improvement & Disparities (2022) *COVID-19: Mental Health and Wellbeing Surveillance Report*. London: HM government. https://www.gov.uk/government/publications/covid-19-mental-health-and-wellbeing-surveillance-report/2-important-findings-so-far

Office for National Statistics (2017) *Changes in the Value and Division of Unpaid Care Work in the UK: 2000 to 2015*. https://www.ons.gov.uk/economy/nationalaccounts/satelliteaccounts/articles/changesinthevalueanddivisionofunpaidcareworkintheuk/2015

Office for National Statistics (2019) *How Would You Support Our Ageing Population?* https://www.ons.gov.uk/peoplepopulationandcommunity/birthsdeathsandmarriages/ageing/articles/howwouldyousupportourageingpopulation/2019-06-24

Office for National Statistics (2020a) *Living Longer: Implications of Childlessness Among Tomorrow's Older Population*. https://www.ons.gov.uk/peoplepopulationandcommunity/birthsdeathsandmarriages/ageing/articles/livinglonger/implicationsofchildlessnessamongtomorrowsolderpopulation

Office for National Statistics (2020b) *Coronavirus and the Social Impacts on Great Britain*. https://www.ons.gov.uk/peoplepopulationandcommunity/healthandsocialcare/healthandwellbeing/datasets/coronavirusandthesocialimpactsongreatbritaindata

References

Office for National Statistics (2022) *People Aged 65 Years and Over in Employment*. https://www.ons.gov.uk/employmentandlabourmarket/peopleinwork/employmentandemployeetypes/articles/peopleaged65yearsandoverinemploymentuk/januarytomarch2022toapriltojune2022

Office for National Statistics (2023a) *Care Homes and Estimating the Self-funding Population, England: 2022 to 2023*. https://www.ons.gov.uk/peoplepopulationandcommunity/healthandsocialcare/socialcare/articles/carehomesandestimatingtheselffundingpopulationengland/2022to2023

Office for National Statistics (2023b) *Average Household Income, UK: Financial Year Ending 2022*. https://www.ons.gov.uk/peoplepopulationandcommunity/personalandhouseholdfinances/incomeandwealth/bulletins/householddisposableincomeandinequality/financialyearending2022

Office for National Statistics (2024) *Childbearing for Women Born in Different Years*. https://www.ons.gov.uk/peoplepopulationandcommunity/birthsdeathsandmarriages/conceptionandfertilityrates/bulletins/childbearingforwomenbornindifferentyearsenglandandwales/

Oldfield, Z., Rogers, N., Phelps, A., Blake, M., Steptoe, A., Oskala, A., et al (2020) *English Longitudinal Study of Ageing: Waves 0–9, 1998–2019*; 33rd Edition. UK Data Service. SN: 5050. http://doi.org/10.5255/UKDA-SN-5050-20 (data files for Wave 9 were used for this book).

Oung, C. (2020) *Social Care Across the Four Countries of the UK: What Can We Learn?* London: Nuffield Trust. https://www.nuffieldtrust.org.uk/news-item/social-care-across-the-four-countries-of-the-uk-what-can-we-learn#lesson-3-create-a-clear-offer

Ovseiko, P. (2007) *Long Term Care for Older People: Age Horizons Brief*. Oxford: HSBC/Oxford Institute of Ageing.

Palmer, R., Turner, G. and Hebden, P. (2019) *A Manifesto for Tax Equality*. London: Tax Justice UK.

Parliamentary Office of Science and Technology (2018) *Postnote 582: Unpaid Care*. London: Parliamentary Office of Science and Technology. http://researchbriefings.files.parliament.uk/documents/POST-PN-0582/POST-PN-0582.pdf&ved=2ahUKEwjA8Ka_w5qFAxVdQUEAHfi-A40QFnoECCIQAQ

Petrie, K. and Kirkup, J. (2018) *Caring for Carers: The Lives of Family Carers in the UK*. London: Age UK.

Petrillo, M. and Bennett, M. (2023) *Valuing Carers 2021: England and Wales*. London: Carers UK with Centre for Care. https://centreforcare.ac.uk/updates/2023/05/valuing-carers/

Pickard, L. (2002) 'The decline of intensive inter-generational care of older people in Great Britain, 1985–1995', *Population Trends*, 110: 31–40.

Pickard, L. (2015) 'A growing care gap? The supply of unpaid care for older people by their adult children in England to 2032', *Ageing & Society*, 35(1): 96–123.

Piepsna-Samarasinha, L. (2018) *Care Work: Dreaming Disability Justice*. Vancouver: Arsenal Pulp Press.

Pollock, A. (2021) 'Multinational care companies are the real winners from Johnson's new tax', *The Guardian*, 14 September. https://www.theguardian.com/commentisfree/2021/sep/14/multinational-care-companies-new-tax-privatised

Preston, J. and Firth, R. (2020) *Coronavirus, Class and Mutual Aid in the United Kingdom*. Cham: Palgrave. https://doi.org/10.1007/978-3-030-57714-8

Public Accounts Committee, House of Commons (2024) *Reforming Adult Social Care in England*. London: House of Commons. https://publications.parliament.uk/pa/cm5804/cmselect/cmpubacc/427/report.html

Public Health Wales (2019) *Making a Difference: Housing and Health: A Care for Investment*. Cardiff: Public Health Wales. https://phwwhocc.co.uk/wp-content/uploads/2020/07/PHW-Making-a-Difference-Housing-and-Health-A-Case-for-Investment-Executive-Summary.pdf

Quilter-Pinner, H. and Hochlaf, D. (2019) *Social Care: Free at the Point of Need –the Case for Free Personal Care in England*. London: Institute for Public Policy Research. http://www.ippr.org/research/publications/social-care-free-at-the-point-of-need

Renaisi (2019) *North and South London Cares; Evaluation and Development through the Centre for Social Action Innovation Fund*. London: North London Cares. https://northlondoncares.org.uk/publications-reports

References

Rochdale Circle (nd) *Making a Difference: Evaluation and Monitoring Report*. Rochdale: Rochdale Circle. https://hmrcircle.org.uk/download/30/making-a-difference-evaluation-amp-amp-monitoring-report

Rocks, S., Boccarini, G., Charlesworth, A., Idriss, O., McConkey, R. and Rachet-Jacquet, L. (2021) *Health and Social Care Funding Projections 2021*. Health Foundation. London: Policy in Practice. https://doi.org/10.37829/HF-2021-RC18

Ross, C.E., Mirowsky, J. and Pribesh, S. (2001) 'Powerlessness and the amplification of threat: Neighborhood disadvantage, disorder, and mistrust', *American Sociological Review*, 66(4): 568–91. https://doi.org/10.2307/3088923

Rowlands, J. (2023) 'Autumn statement 2023: uprating benefits: the long view', *Policy in Practice* blog, https://policyinpractice.co.uk/autumn-statement-2023-uprating-benefits-the-long-view/

Ryan-Collins, J., Stephens, L. and Coote, A. (2008) *The New Wealth of Time: How Timebanking Helps People Build Better Public Services*. London: New Economics Foundation.

Sabey, A., Seers, H., Chatterjee, H.J. and Polley, M. (2022) *How Can Social Prescribing Support Older People in Poverty? A Rapid Scoping Review of Interventions*. London: University College London. https://www.ucl.ac.uk/biosciences/culture-nature-health-research/social-prescribing

Samuel, M. (2022a) 'Social care waiting lists up 37% in 6 months, finds ADASS', *Community Care*, 4 August. https://www.communitycare.co.uk/2022/08/04/social-care-waiting-lists-up-37-in-6-months-finds-adass/

Samuel, M. (2022b) 'Three-quarters of large councils planning to tighten eligibility for adult social care, finds survey', *Community Care*, 11 November. https://www.communitycare.co.uk/2022/11/11/three-quarters-of-large-councils-planning-to-tighten-eligibility-for-adult-social-care-finds-survey/

Samuel, M. (2023) 'Councils rationing adult social care through "subjective" eligibility judgments, finds think-tank', *Community Care*, 5 November. https://www.communitycare.co.uk/2023/11/05/councils-rationing-adult-social-care-through-subjective-eligibility-judgments-finds-think-tank/

Samuel, M. (2024) 'Worst financial outlook for years for adult social care revealed by directors' survey', *Community Care*, 16 July. https://www.communitycare.co.uk/2024/07/19/overseas-recruitment-drives-latest-growth-in-adult-social-care-workforce/

Scharf, T. and de Jong Gierveld, J. (2008) Loneliness in urban neighbourhoods: an Anglo-Dutch comparison. *European Journal of Ageing*, 5: 103–15.

Scottish Government (2019a) *Social Care Report*. Edinburgh: Scottish Government.

Scottish Government (2019b) *Scottish Social Care Survey*. Edinburgh: Scottish Government.

Scottish Government (2021) *Care Homes for Adults in Scotland: Statistics for 2011–2021*. Edinburgh: Scottish Government. https://publichealthscotland.scot/publications/care-home-census-for-adults-in-scotland/care-home-census-for-adults-in-scotland-statistics-for-2011-to-2021-full-release/

Scottish Government (2022) *Free Personal and Nursing Care in Scotland, 2020/21*. Edinburgh: Scottish Government. https://www.gov.scot/publications/free-personal-nursing-care-scotland-2020-21/pages/2/

Scottish Government Health and Social Care (2021) *People Who Access Social Care and Unpaid Carers in Scotland*. Edinburgh: Scottish Government. https://tinyurl.com/5y6xue54

Scottish Trades Union Congress (2022) *Profiting from Care: Why Scotland Can't Afford Privatised Social Care*. https://www.stuc.org.uk/resources/profiting-from-care-report.pdf

Scottish Women's Budget Group (2023) *Towards a Transformative Adult Social Care Support Service for Scotland*. https://www.swbg.org.uk/content/publications/Towards-a-transformative-universal-adult-social-care-support-service-for-Scotland.pdf

Segal, L. (2023) *Lean on Me: A Politics of Radical Care*. London: Verso.

Sheffield Hallam University (2022) *Leeds Neighbourhood Network Phase 2 Evaluation*. London: Centre for Ageing Better. https://ageing-better.org.uk/resources/leeds-neighbourhood-network-phase-two

References

Sikka, P. (2023) 'What the autumn statement will deliver, and what Jeremy Hunt will do instead', *Left Foot Forward*, 17 November. https://leftfootforward.org/2023/11/what-the-autumn-statement-should-deliver-and-what-jeremy-hunt-will-do-instead/

Singh, S. (2017) *The Evolution of Giving: An Exploration of Time Banking as a Community Development Instrument*. South Carolina Honors College, Senior Theses, 188. https://scholarcommons.sc.edu/senior_theses/188

Sitrin, M. and Colectiva Sembrar (eds) (2020) *Pandemic Solidarity: Mutual Aid during the Covid-19 Crisis*. London: Pluto Press.

Skills for Care (2018) *The Economic Value of the Adult Social Care Sector*. London: Skills for Care. https://www.skillsforcare.org.uk/About-us/Skills-for-Care-and-Development/Economic-value-of-the-adult-social-care-sector.aspx

Skills for Care (2023) *Adult Social Care Workforce Estimates 2022/23*. London: Skills for Care. https://www.skillsforcare.org.uk/Adult-Social-Care-Workforce-Data/Workforce-intelligence/publications/national-information/The-state-of-the-adult-social-care-sector-and-workforce-in-England.aspx

Social Exclusion Unit (2006) *A Sure Start to Later Life: Ending Inequalities for Older People*. London: Office of the Deputy Prime Minister.

Social Work Scotland (2020) *Adult Social Care Expenditure in the Decade of Austerity – Scotland Compared with Rest of U.K.* Edinburgh: Social Work Scotland. https://socialworkscotland.org/wp-content/uploads/2020/11/SWS-Supp-Sub-2-ASC-EXPENDITURE-IN-THE-DECADE-OF-AUSTERITY.pdf

Spade, D. (2020) *Mutual Aid: Building Solidarity During This Crisis (and the Next)*. London: Verso Press. https://theanarchistlibrary.org/library/dean-spade-mutual-aid

Spinelli, G., Weaver, P., Marks, M. and Victor, C. (2019) 'Making a case for creating living labs for aging-in-place: enabling socially innovative models for experimentation and complementary economies', *Frontiers in Sociology*, 4(19). Doi: 10.3389/fsoc.2019.00019.

Sturrock, D. and Tallack, C. (2022) *Does the Cap Fit? Analysing the Government's Proposed Amendment to the English Social Care Charging System*. London: Institute for Fiscal Studies. https://ifs.org.uk/publications/does-cap-fit-analysing-governments-proposed-amendment-english-social-care-charging

Sutherland, A. (2017) 'Review of Peter Limbrick, "Caring Activism"', *Disability and Society*, 32(4): 608–10. Doi: 10.1080/09687599.2017.1294389.

Tiratelli, L. and Kaye, S. (2020) *Communities vs Coronavirus; The Rise of Mutual Aid*. London: New Local (formerly the New Local Government Network). www.newlocal.org.uk

Tronto, J.C. (2005) 'An ethic of care', in Cudd, A.E. and Andreasen, R.O. (eds) *Feminist Theory: A Philosophical Anthology*. Oxford: Blackwell, pp 251–69.

Tronto, J.C. (2013) *Caring Democracy: Markets, Equality, and Justice*. New York: New York University Press.

UKHCA (UK Home Care Association) (2021) *An Overview of the UK Homecare Market*. Wellington: UKHCA. https://www.homecareassociation.org.uk/resource/market-overview-2021.html

UKHCA (UK Home Care Association) (2023) *A Minimum Price for Homecare*. London: UKHCA. https://www.homecareassociation.org.uk/static/e1b6e23b-7f3e-48bd-be2027305e5b40c9/Homecare-Association-Minimum-Price-for-Homecare-England-2024-2025.pdf

Van Baarsen, B. (2002) 'Theories on coping with loss: the impact of social support and self-esteem on adjustment to emotional and social loneliness following a partner's death in later life', *Journals of Gerontology: Psychological Sciences and Social Sciences*, 57B(1): S33–42.

Walker, C.C. (2021) 'Predatory financial tactics are putting the very survival of the UK care system at risk', *The Guardian*, 10 August. https://www.theguardian.com/commentisfree/2021/aug/10/predatory-financial-tactics-survival-uk-care-system-at-risk

Wang, X. (2023) 'How to develop the time bank for old-age service in less developed areas: a comparison of Nanning and Nanjing', *Highlights in Business, Economics and Management*, 8: 488–94. Doi: 10.54097/hbem.v8i.7259.

Wanless, D. (2006) *Securing Good Care for Older People*. London: King's Fund.

Wein, T. (2020) *New Solidarity: How Mutual Aid Might Change Britain*. Devizes: The Dignity Project. www.dignityproject.net

References

Welsh Government (2023) *Towards a National Care and Support Service for Wales: Initial Implementation Plan*. Cardiff: Welsh Government. https://www.gov.wales/sites/default/files/publications/2023-12/Towards%2520a%2520National%2520Care%2520and%2520Support%2520Service%2520initial%2520implementation%2520plan.pdf

Welsh National Commissioning Board (2017) *Outcomes-Based Home Care Commissioning Toolkit: Commissioning for Outcomes in Social Care*. Cardiff: Welsh National Commissioning Board. https://www.wlga.wales/introduction-to-the-home-care-toolkit

Wenger, C. (1994) *Understanding Support Networks and Community Care*. Aldershot: Avebury.

Wenger, G.C., Davies, R., Shahtahmasebi, S. and Scott, A. (1996) 'Social isolation and loneliness in old age', *Ageing and Society*, 16(3): 333–58.

Wernham, T. and Brewer, M. (2022) *Income and Wealth Inequality Explained in Five Charts*. London: Institute for Fiscal Studies. https://ifs.org.uk/articles/income-and-wealth-inequality-explained-5-charts

West, D. (2024) 'Exclusive: social care waiting times revealed for first time in a decade', *Health Service Journal*, 25 March. https://www.hsj.co.uk/integrated-care/exclusive-social-care-waiting-times-revealed-for-first-time-in-a-decade/7036852.article

Westhall, A. and Hughes, C. (2019) *Social Care Innovation by the Social Economy in Manchester, Greater Manchester and the North of England*. Manchester: Manchester University with Joseph Rowntree Foundation. https://www.research.manchester.ac.uk/files/156367701/IGAU_Briefing_11_Social_Care_Innovation_3.pdfandved=2ahUKEwjr8pfZv4iFAxWeW0EAHf-uDp4QFnoECA8QAQandusg=AOvVaw3vvlmvvuzvkw1qYOUOsOpQ

Whitty, C. (2023) *Chief Medical Officer's Annual Report 2023: Health in an Ageing Society*. London: Department of Health and Social Care. https://www.gov.uk/government/publications/chief-medical-officers-annual-report-2023-health-in-an-ageing-society

WHO (World Health Organization) (2024) *The WHO Age-Friendly Cities Framework*. Geneva: WHO. https://extranet.who.int/agefriendlyworld/age-friendly-cities-framework/

Wilson, J.V. (2015) *Time Eases All Things: A Critical Study of How Time Banks Attempt to Use Time-Based Currency to Alleviate Social Exclusion*. Salford: University of Salford, School of Nursing, Midwifery, Social Work and Social Sciences, PhD thesis. https://salford-repository.worktribe.com/output/1407130/time-eases-all-things-a-critical-study-of-how-time-banks-attempt-to-use-time-based-currency-to-alleviate-social-exclusion

Women's Budget Group (2020) *Creating a Caring Economy: A Call to Action*. London: WBG.

Woodard, K. (2015) 'Britain's fear of growing old alone', *Express*, 11 July. https://www.express.co.uk/comment/expresscomment/590479/Britain-fear-growing-old-alone

Zigante, V., Fernandez, J. and Mazzotta, F. (2021) 'Changes in the balance between formal and informal care supply in England between 2001 and 2011: evidence from census data', *Health Economics, Policy and Law*, 16(2): 232–49. Doi: https://doi.org/10.1017/S1744133120000146.

Index

References to figures appear in *italic* type; those in **bold** type refer to tables.

A

ACORN community union 7, 133–4, 170
'activities of daily living' (ADLs) 35–6, 57, 68, 72, 143
ADL/IADL difficulties **35**, 37, 39–40, 43, 45, 46–7
adult children 34, 46, **182**
Adult Social Care Funding Pressures (Health Foundation) 81
advocacy 103
Age Friendly City (Manchester) 146
'age-friendly communities' 9, 10, 145–7, 152, 155, 161, 171, *172*
age-friendly transport strategies 147
Ageing Well Without Children 50
Age UK 36, 72, 112, 139, 146, 150
aging 44–6
Alderwick, H. 73
Aldridge, H. 32
Allan, Thomas 98–9
anchor organisations 85, 141
arts-based approaches 100
assessments
 Care Act 2014 33–5, 96
 Scotland 60
 waiting lists 28, 61, 72–3, 102
Association of Directors of Adult Social Services (ADASS) 28, 61, 69
Attendance Allowance 65, 82, 165

B

Barnet, North London 146
bathrooms and bathroom assistance 104, 151, 178, **179**
Be Caring (Newcastle) 86–7

bedroom assistance 104, **179**
befriending schemes 109–10, 125, 169–70
Bell, D. 58, 59, 80
'Big Society' agenda 119, 128–9, 141
Birkbeck University 100
Black Lives Matter 122, 124
Black Panthers 123
Blood, I. 111
Brighton 134
Brimblecombe, N. 30–1, 45
Bristol 122, 133, 134
British Household Panel Survey 53, 54, 57, 58–9, 108–9
Buurtzorg model 88, 154

C

Cahn, Edgar 126, 127
Callaghan, L. 111
Cambridge County Council 85
Cameron government 119, 128–9
Campsbourne Community Collective 95, 99–103, 116, 125
Canada 63, 122
care
 defining 16–17
 demand for 14, 44, 89–90
 and gender 43
 qualitative aspects 7, 94
 quantitative aspects 94
 reducing need for 10, 143–58, 171
 severe needs 74, 79, 116
 shortage 44
Care Act 2014 33, 35, 37, 71, 74, 151
Care Act assessments 33–5, 96
care activism 141–2, 170

care agencies 77
care as a relationship 6–7, 96–7, 166–7, 167–8
'Care as Commons' (Allan) 98–9
care budgets
 cuts 11–14, 140
 deficits 5
 increases needed 65, 81–2
 labour costs 76
 NEF/WBG 74–80
 working-age disabled people 14
care charges 92–3
care cost cap proposals
 lifetime cap 14, 70, 163–4
 weekly cap 120, 163
Care Collective 2–3, 6, 96–8, 106, 115–16, 120–1, 123–4, 141
care cooperatives 85–7, 165
care deficits 41, 44–6, 47
Care England 76–7
care ethics 98
care homes *see* residential care
care needs 34–8
Care Policy and Evaluation Centre (CPEC, LSE) 44–5, 74
Care Professional Academy 85
Care Quality Commission 84–5
carer burnout 61
care reforms 67, 79, 91
carers, formal
 see care workforce
carers, informal
 ages 23, 30, 46
 and COVID–19 pandemic 26–7, **27**, 55
 digital exclusion 148
 emotional impact 103
 gender 43
 isolation 108
 mental and physical health 32
 numbers of 23
 poverty 32, 103
 qualities 102
 support for 60–2, 81–2, 160, 164–5
 see also informal carers
Carer's Allowance 4, 64–5, 66, 81–2, 160, 165
carer's leave 61–2, 63, 165
Carer's Leave Act 2023 62
carer stress 25, 31–2, 43, 60, 61, 160
Carers UK 17, 24, 27, 31
Cares Family 115, 116, 168

care tasks 103, 104–5
'care team' approaches 88, 154
care workforce 14, 16
 growth 20
 pay 73, 75–9, 83, 91, 162
 unfilled vacancies 76
'caring community' 96–7, 120
'caring economy' 10, 94–117, 160, 168
 Care Collective 2–3, 6, 7
 Circles projects 111–15
 elements of 99
 informal care 104–5
 loneliness 106–11
 as a relationship 96–7
 universal care service 173
'caring society' 168
Carmichael, F. 54–5
Carrino, L. 54
cash allowances 63–4, 81–2
Cattell, V. 107–8
Censuses for England and Wales 2011 and 2021 18, 20–6, **26**, 28, 29–30, 47
Centre for Ageing Better 145
Chan, T. 50
charities 138
Chatzidikis, A. 96–7, 106, 120–1
Chief Medical Officer's Annual Report 2023 (Whitty) 144
childlessness 38–9, 41, 47–50, **50**, 53, 106
children 23, 31, 38–41, 46, 50–3
Children's Society 23
China 131, 132
Circles projects 85–6, 111–15, 168
close friends 106, 107
collective agency for change 120
collective projects 140
'commons of care' 97–103, 123–4, 142, 160, 168, 173
Community Action Tenants Union (Northern Ireland) 133
community-based co-productions 86
'community care' services 57
Community Catalysts 83–4, 85, 138
community centres 145–6, 148
community development workers 157
community informants 166
Community Interest Companies 87, 138, 140

Index

community messaging 124–5
Community Microenterprises 137
community projects 7, 99–100, 116, 153, 171, **172**
community solidarity 66, 137–9, 141, 146, 161, 167–71, 183
community stability 110
community unions 133–4, 141–2, 170
continuous care 21
cooperatives 92
Cooper, B. 5–6, 17, 69
co-production of care services 10, 127, 169
Cornwall 153
cost estimates
  care reform 4–6
  free care 68–9, 80–1
  help for unpaid carers 81–2
  homecare **176–7**
  'outcomes-based commissioning' 87–8
  proposals 89–93
  residential care 88–9, **177**
  supply-side changes 83, 92, 165–6
  universal care service 68, 73–80
Cottam, Hilary 111–12, 168
council-commissioned care 19, **19**
Council for Voluntary Service 138
Council Tax 149
County Councils Network 13
COVID-19 pandemic 13, 21
  carer stress 61
  community solidarity 137
  Haringey Circle 114
  informal care 25, 26–7, **27**, 55
  and mental health 31
  mutual aid groups (MAGs) 97, 118, 119–25, 141, 170–1
  NHS Volunteer Responders 134–5, 170–1
  Scotland 59

D

Darton, R., 111
daughters 32, 39–40, **39**, 46–7, 49–50, 55, 104
day centres **19**, 56, 140
'decade of austerity' 21, 25
de Jong Gierveld, J. 107
demand for care 44, 89–90
dementia 95, 143
demographic trends 3, 25, 44–8
Demos 153

Denmark 62–3, 64, 78, 82
Department of Health and Social Care 136
depression 107
Derbyshire 153
diet 149
'digital champions' 148
digital exclusion 148–9
digital skills support 7, 37–8, 148–9, 167
dignity 37
disability benefits 102
Disability Facilities Grant 151
disabled adult children 30, 42
disabled adults 46, 50, 51–2, 65
disabled children 24, 31, 52, 102–3
Disabled People Against Cuts (DPAC) 82
Disclosure and Barring Service (DBS) 103, 138, 157
diverse social networks 106, 183–90
divorce 50
Doing it Right (Somerset County Council) 84
Dowling, E. 6
Dubb, S. 127

E

early-stage impairments 144
education 50–1
eldercare 15, 25, 32, 46, 49, 145
Elfrida (interviewee) 62, 106, 184–5
emotional support 6–7, 95, 96, 99, 101, 103, 106–7, 166
End Social Care Disgrace 65, 81, 103
England
  ACORN community union 133–4
  assessment waiting lists 73
  care reform 67
  'community care' services 57
  council bankruptcies 67–8
  FPC for seniors 80–1
  means test thresholds 70
  over-75s living alone 47
  population of over-65s 25
  social enterprises 169
  spending per head 162
  tax revenues 163, 174, **175–7**
  value of care sector **19**
English Longitudinal Study of Ageing (ELSA) Wave 9, 11, 16, 20–1, 69
  ADL/IADL difficulties 39–40

food shopping 37
informal 'personal' care 18
loneliness 37
need for help by age 104, 178, **179**
partner care for over-65's 38
unmet needs 36, 72
Equal Care Coop 85–6, 154
Ermisch, J. 50
Essex County Council 137–8
Essex Wellbeing Service 137
'excluded' networks 108
exercise 149
extra-care housing 5, 89, 152

F

Fabian Society 5–6, 17, 69, 70–1
Fair Shares (Gloucestershire) 130, 132
family carers 3–4, 13, 28, 52, 82
Family Resources Survey
   (FRS) 11, 20–1
  carers over 65, 46
  defining caring roles 24
  hours caring 26
  informal care 21, 22, 27–8, 32
  intensification of care 28
  non-relatives as carers 40
  unpaid care 31
fear of crime 110
feminist ethics of care 98
Finland 64
focus groups 186–90
food banks 125
food insecurity 148
formal care 3
  defining 15
  demand for 44
  making affordable 9
  marketising 98–9
  negotiating 103
  NHS savings and taxes 91
  partnership status 32–4, **35**
  and personal care 97, 142, 167
  reducing costs 165–6
  reducing need for 8–9, 112, 173
  and reduction in loneliness 115
  scale of 17–20
  substitution debate 55–60
  workers' pay 159–60
  see also informal care
formal group activities 109
formal homecare
  capacity of the care system 72
  FPC in Scotland 75

NEF/WBG scenario 81
outcome-based commissioning 153
over-65s in England 13–14
'personal budget' 63
'relational care' and agency staff 166
task-oriented 96
'Frailty' 15
France 63
free care 6, 68, 71–2, 80–1, 92,
   159, 164
'free homecare' (Tower Hamlets) 15
free personal care (FPC) 5
  cost estimates 80–1
  defining 17, 57, 68
  and informal care 57–9
  residential care 58, 80
  Scotland 17, 43, 55–7, 162–3
  underfunding 59–60
free training 85
free universal care 9, 159, 173
friends
  continuity of contact 109
  decline in contribution 53
  emotional support 95, 106
  as 'family' of childless 48–9
  informal care **39**, 104–5
  intimate care 139
  loneliness 107
  natural contacts 116
  offering help 40
  sources of support 95
  see also neighbours
friendship networks 53, 149, 168
fuel poverty 148, 153
full-time equivalent homecare 78–9
future care demand 4, 42
  ageing population 44–7
  childlessness 47–51
  disabilities 51–2
  informal care 60–1
  and non-relatives 52–3
  trends in supply and demand 43
future cost of care 78–80, 161–3

G

gardening and garden
   maintenance 3, 17, 35, 37
gay community 106, 123
General Household Survey 46, 53
Generation Exchange (Haringey and
   Enfield) 149
Generations Working Together
   (Scotland) 148

Index

Germany 63–4
Give&Take Care 132
'good neighbour' schemes 111
Gostoli, U. 51
gradient of intimacy 104
Graeber, David 99
Gray, C. 126, 127
Green, H. 53
Grey Matters Productions
    (Brighton) 149

H

Hammersmith and Fulham
    Council 15, 71–2, 75–6, 80
Hanover Housing Group 111
Haringey Circle 113–14, 156
Haringey, London 99–100, 124–5
Harrop, A. 5–6, 17, 69
Hayashi, M. 129
health advice 8–9, 44, 143, 149–50
health and care services 147–8
Health Foundation 65, 70, 73, 74,
    81, 90
Health Survey of England (HSE) 11,
    20–1, 69, 178
    ADL difficulties 43, 46, 72
    age of partners as carers 38
    formal homecare 13–14
    help with tasks 180, **181**
    homecare 37
    informal care **182**
    over-65s needing help 26
    self-funded care 16
    support for carers 61
    unmet needs 36, **36**, 104, **179**
healthy life expectancy 9, 44,
    143–4, 150
'heterogeneous' networks 108
Heywood, Middleton and
    Rochdale Circle 7, 111, 113,
    116, 156
higher education 50–1
Hochlaf, D. 79, 81, 82
homecare
    abolishing charges 71–2
    cost savings 165–6
    demand for 18, 91
    and personal care 167
    reducing costs 83
    subsidies 70
    value **19**
    workforce 18, 19, **20**
    zero-hours contracts 76

homes and housing 151–3
    adaptations and repairs 151,
    158, 166
    designing 110, 145, 151
    extra-care housing 20, 89, 152
    exchange system 158
    and healthcare services 153
    maintenance 7, 37
'homogeneous' networks 108
'hotel costs' of residential care 58, 78
'household satellite accounts'
    (ONS) 17
housework 57
Housing Benefit 149
Hu, B. 45
Hughes, F. 32
Hull and East Riding
    Timebank 127, 130
'hunger march' (September
    2023) 125
Hurricane Katrina 126, 133
Hyacinth (interviewee) 50, 51,
    106, 183–4

I

'impaired' adults 52
Industrial Workers of the World 120
informal care 3, 160–1
    childlessness 47–51
    community solidarity projects 7
    community support 159, 160
    COVID-19 pandemic 26–8
    defining 15, 21
    demographic trends 44
    dependence on 160
    and formal care 17, 32–4
    and FPC 57–60
    friends and neighbours 104–5
    intensification of care 28–31, *29*
    and mutual aid 96–7
    partnership status 32–4, **35**
    providers and relationships 38–40, **39**
    scale of 16, 17–20
    shortage of care 44
    substitution debate 55–60
    supply and demand 43, 44–5
    survey questions 22–3
    sustaining 10, 66
    trends 25–8, **26**, 27
    types of help and helpers **181**
    women 42–3
    younger people 31
    see also formal care

informal carers
　assessment of needs 33–4
　childless singles 38–9
　employment and pensions 32, 53–4, 61–4
　estimates of numbers 18, 20–5
　and free personal care 58
　growing need for 10
　help for 81–2, 90
　long hours 57
　needs 34, 99–100
　new policies 60–5
　recognition and encouragement 65
　remuneration 5, 81–2
　role of partners 33–5, 38, 39, 45–7, 97, 103
　shortfall 43, 45
　supporting 139–40, 164–5
　trends 25–6, **26**, *27*, **182**
　of working age 31–2
　(*see also* carers, informal)
Institute for Public Policy Research (IPPR) 79, 81, 82
Institute of Community Studies 100
'instrumental activities of daily living' (IADLs) 35–6, 105
　see also ADL/IADL difficulties
intensification of care 13, 28–31, *29*, 46
intensive carers 60, 65, 95, 121, 165
intergenerational contacts 110–11, 114–15, 148–9
the internet 37–8, 150
interviews 102, 183–90
intimate care 131, 139, 178–80, **179**, **181**
isolation 17, 37, 95, 108, 116, 147–8
Italy 63

J

Japan 128–9, 131, 132
Jo (interviewee) 30, 52, 60, 103, 183, 186

K

Karlsberg-Schaffer, S. 58
Kartupelis, J. 96, 97, 98–9, 166
Keser, Burçu (Bu) 101, 185–6
Kirkup, J. 46

L

Labour Force Survey 54
Laing-Buisson report 17–18

'LA needs' (NEF/WBG) 74–5, 78, 78–9, 81
Lebanon 122
Leeds 134
Leeds Neighbourhood Networks 116, 155–7, 168, 170
Lewisham Local 131
LGBTQIA+ 106, 123
life expectancy 45
　healthy life expectancy 9, 40, 143–4
'lifetime care cost cap' 70
Limbrick, P. 154, 170
'linking' social capital 106
Living Rent (Scotland) 133
Living Wage Foundation 76
Li, Y. 108–9
lobbying 147
local authorities
　age groups' needs 14
　annual budgets 25, 90
　care agencies' rates 76
　carers' wages 77
　homecare labour force 19, **20**
　and MAG 123
　residential care fees 89
　shortage of care 13
　social care spending 17, 19, 25
London boroughs viii, 5, 71, 147
London Borough of Camden 111
London Borough of Hammersmith and Fulham 15, 71–2, 75–6, 80
London Borough of Haringey 124
London Borough of Southwark 111
London Borough of Tower Hamlets 15, 71–2
'London Loos' (Age UK) 147
London School of Economics and Political Science (LSE) 44–5, 74
loneliness 17
　'age-friendly communities' 145
　alleviating for preserving health 116
　community projects 116
　coronary heart disease 95
　and formal care 35
　and 'neighbours' 115
　personal networks 106–11
　psychological wellbeing 37, 107
　reducing 147–8
long-term health conditions 51–2
'Love My Neighbour' initiative 114

Index

lunch clubs 7, 118, 119, 140
Lunt, N. 119

M

Maher, J. 53
managing paperwork 105
Manchester 86, 146–7, 152, 155
Manchester Older People's
  Network 155
Margaret (interviewee) 48–9, 106
Mayo, M. 123
McNamee, P. 58, 59
means testing 13, 18–19, 68, 70
men 38, 45, 47, 54
mental stimulation 95
micro-enterprises 83–5, 92,
  138–9, 165
minimum homecare wage
  (UKHCA) 77
Minimum Income Guarantee 64
minor impairments 144
mobility 189–90
mothers 32, 42, 102
Mowat, David 49
mutual aid 118–19, 170, 173
  'co-optation' by state 123
  COVID-19 pandemic 170–1
  and informal care 96–7
  international movement 122
  between neighbours 128, 183–90
  reciprocity and co-production 169
  sheltered housing 186–90
  and 'solidarity' 8, 99
  state as neglectful 123
  and timebanks 126
mutual aid groups (MAGs) 99–100,
  118–25, 169
  Care Collective 120–1
  COVID-19 pandemic 97, 118,
    119–25, 141, 170–1
  funding 141
  Haringey 124–5
  middle class members 136–7
  political role 122–3
  and timebanks 136–7, 140
  United States 122–3
  WhatsApp 124–5
mutuality 99

N

Nanjing, China 131
National Academy of Social
  Prescribing 148

National Audit Office (NAO) 17, 77
national care service 2, 5
National Living Wage (NLW) 74,
  75, 76, 77, 81
'neighbourhood attachment' index
  (Li) 108–9
Neighbourhood Cares Pilot
  (Cambridgeshire) 154
Neighbourhood Networks 155–8
neighbours **39**, 40, 53, 104–11,
  121, 139
  see also friends
'network supported housing
  schemes' 152
network theory 7, 106
Newcastle 86–7
New Economics Foundation
  and Women's Budget Group
  (NEF/WBG) 73–5, 77–9, 81,
  81–2, 161–2, 174–7
New Orleans 126, 133
New York 131
New Zealand 126
NHS 17, 91, 147
NHS England 149
NHS Volunteer Responders
  119–20, 134–6, 142, 170
non-family/non-relatives 6
  and the gradient of intimacy 104
  home and garden maintenance 7
  instrumental activities 105, 167
  safety-critical tasks 139–40
  social care 120
  support for single and childless 168
  support from 6, 39, 40, 52–3
'non-personal' care 56, 59
non-profit enterprises 7
non-profit formal care 97
non-profit residential care 89
'Nordic' option (NEF/WBG) 78
Northern Ireland 23, 70, 133, 162
North London Cares 7, 114–15
North West Care Cooperative -
  Chester 87, 92
North Yorkshire 153
Norway 63
Nottingham Circle 112–13
nursing care **19**

O

Office for National Statistics
  (ONS) 17
offsetting savings 79–80

225

Open University 100
Organisation for Economic
 Co-operation and
 Development 63
'outcome-based commissioning'
 87–8, 153–5, 165–6, 169–70
over-50s clubs 111
over-65s
 with ADL/IADL difficulties 40
 with 'LA need' 79
 living alone 47, *48*
 partner care 38
 supported by social care 15
 UK population 44
over-75s living alone 47
over-85s relying on children 47–8
owner-occupiers 110

P

Pannell, J. 111
parents 40, 50
partners 33, 38–9, **39**, 46–7
'Partners in Care' (Maryland) 131–2
Patel, Pragna 98
pay 68–9, 75–8
 see also wage costs
paying bills 105
peer support groups 132, 149
personal budgets **19**, 69, 71, 82, 92
'personal care' 5–6
 costs of free care 80
 defining 16–17, 104
 and formal care 97, 167
 and informal care 21
 Scotland 68, 69, 91
Personal Independence
 Payment 102
'personalisation' of care 138
personal networks 106–11
Personal Social Services Research
 Unit (LSE) 44, 65
Petrie, K. 46
'politics of compassion' 94, 97–103
poor health 37, 54–5, 107
PossAbilities C.I.C. 87
poverty 37, 54–5, 150–1
preventive health measures 9, 44,
 80, 92, 95, 144–5, 149–50, 171
privacy and family autonomy 104–5
privately funded care *see* residential
 care; self-funded care
'propensity to care' 4, 43, 45–6, 51,
 65, 66

public toilets 147
public transport 154
Puerto Rican communities 123

Q

quality of care 88, 153–5
quality of life 95, 144, 153
Quilter-Pinner, H. 79, 81, 82

R

RadioReverb 149
'rationing' care 56
'Real Living Wage' 76, 77–8
reciprocity 127, 169
'relational care' 96, 97, 166–7
relatives 39, **39**, 54–5, 82, 106
religious organisations 108
residential care 5, **19**, 58–9, 70,
 88–9, 151, 166
 see also self-funded care
residential care workers 75
residents' associations 125
residents' groups 111
respite care 165
retirement ages 3, 54
retirement housing 109, 111
Roar Do Digital (Renfrewshire) 148
Rochdale Borough
 Housing 111, 113
Rochdale Circle 7, 111, 113,
 116, 156
Royal Voluntary Service
 (RVS) 134, 135
Rural Action Derbyshire 148
rural areas 107, 145, 148
Rushey Green timebank 130, 131
Ryan-Collins, J. 131

S

savings 18–19, 112
Scharf, T. 107
Scotland
 adult carers 23
 Buurtzorg model trials 88
 Carer's Allowance 65
 clinical needs 68
 COVID-19 pandemic 59
 formal care 18, 56, 59–60
 free personal care (FPC) 17, 18,
  43, 55–8, 67, 80, 91, 162–3
 informal carers 59, 72
 Living Rent 133
 means test thresholds 70

Index

National Care Service 163
personal care 69
residential care 70, 80
social care spending 57, 162–3
spending and service levels 14
underfunding 56
universal basic income 64
unmet needs 56
Scottish Household Survey 58
Scottish Women's Budget Group 77
Segal, Lynne 6, 96, 98, 99, 101, 115–16
self-funded care 14, 16, 18–19, **19**, 37, 102–3
see also residential care
seniors 15
  ADL difficulties 46
  care packages 73
  children 104
  housing developments 152
  needs 178–82
  networks 155–6
  population 20, 25
  retirement housing estates 109
severe needs 74, 79, 116
'shared lives' 5, 152–3
sheltered housing 140, 152, 186–90
Silverman, E. 51
single seniors 39, 41, 47–8, 106
social activities 68, 95, 109, 130–1, 140, 146, 147, 155
social care 1, 17, 166
social connections 148, 149
social enterprises 140, 165, 169
social inclusion 144, 171
social networks 44, 95, 106, 109, 124, 183–90
'social prescribing' 95, 130–1, 147–8, 149–50
socio-economic groups 51, 52
Soham Community Association 154
'solidaristic' networks 107–8
'solidarity' 8, 120, 136–7, 171
Somerset 84–5
Somerset County Council 84
sons **39**, 46–7, 49–50, 55
South Africa 122
South London Cares 115
Southwark Circle 112, 113
Spade, D. 123
sports clubs 108
staff retention 76
stairs 151, 178, **179**

the state
  mutual aid 122–3
  replacing/enhancing services 119
  and timebanks 128–9
state budgets 5
state pension ages 44–5, 54
'strengths-based commissioning' 155
'subjective eligibility rationing' 73
'substitution debate' 43, 55–60
Suffolk Age UK 139
Suffolk Circle 112–13
Suffolk County Council 137–9
Suffolk Family Carers 112
supportive friendships 7, 96, 109, 111–15
Sutherland, A. 170–1
Sweden 63
Swindon 134

T

tax revenue 5, 80, 91, 163, 174, **175–6**
'Third Way' approaches 129
Thurrock, Essex 85
Timebanking UK 149–50
timebanks 125–32, 140
  community solidarity 141
  financial and leadership basis 136–7
  interpersonal services 131
  as mutual aid 118–19, 125–6, 160–1
  personal networks 129–30
  principles 127
  reciprocity 126, 128, 169
  and the state 128–9
  'take and give' principle 140–1
  transactional principle 126–7
time exchange 130
time-givers 130, 132
'Toilet Manifesto for London' 147
Tower Hamlets 15, 71–2
trades unions 120
The Tribe Project CIC 138
Tronto, J.C. 98
'tuk-tuk' service 154

U

UK Home Care Association (UKHCA) 74, 77, 79, 83
Understanding Society 50, 54
UNISON 76
United States 89, 122–3, 131–2

universal basic income (UBI) 4, 64, 82
universal care service 73
Universal Credit 64
universal free care 68, 163–4
university graduates 50–1
University of the Third Age 113–14
unmet needs 36, **36**, 56, 72–4, 95
unpaid care *see* informal care
unpaid carers *see* informal carers

V

Van Baarsen, B. 109
volunteer exchanges 132
volunteer organisations 139–40, 148
volunteers and voluntary work 15, 85–6, 109, 119–20, 134–5

W

wage costs 73–80, 91
  see also pay
waiting lists 14, 28, 61, 72–3, 102
Wales 14, 25, 47, 67, 70, 107, 162
Wein, T. 122
wellbeing 35, 37
Wenger, C. 107
West London Southall Black Sisters 98
WhatsApp 124–5
wheelchair people 189

Whitty, C. 144
'widening the caring circle' 94–5
'wider needs' 75
widows 43, 47
women
  ADL/IADL difficulties 43
  caring for partners 38
  childlessness 48, **50**
  continuous care 21
  difficulties caring 105
  employment and care 53–4
  living with a partner 47
  responsibility for informal care 42–3
  state pension 54
  without partners 47
Women's Budget Group 6, 73
working-age carers 32
working-age disabled people 14
'work search' obligations 64
World Health Organization (WHO) 145

Y

YouGov 22–3, 24, 27
younger people needing care 31, 51

Z

zero-hours contracts 76

www.ingramcontent.com/pod-product-compliance
Lightning Source LLC
Chambersburg PA
CBHW051538020426
42333CB00016B/1991